NUTRITION IN GENERAL PRACTICE

Edited by Judith Buttriss PhD, SRD

2 Promoting Health and Preventing Disease

SERIES EDITOR: Colin Waine OBE, FRCGP, FRCPath

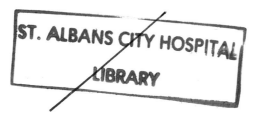
Published by

The Royal College of General Practitioners

1995

The Royal College of General Practitioners was founded in 1952, with this object:

"To encourage, foster and maintain the highest possible standards in general medical practice and for that purpose to take or join with others in taking steps consistent with the charitable nature of that object which may assist towards the same."

Among its responsibilities under its Royal Charter the College is entitled to:

"Diffuse information on all matters affecting general medical practice and issue such publications as may assist the object of the College."

First published by the Exeter Publications Office of the
Royal College of General Practitioners 1995

Typeset by Exe Valley Dataset Ltd., Exeter
Printed by Latimer Trend, Plymouth

ISBN 0 85084 214 X

Contents

Preface to Part 2   ...   .   *v*

Preface to Part 1   ...   .   *vii*

Section 1: The Needs of Specific Age Groups

1. Preconception, pregnancy and lactation   3

2. Infant feeding and weaning   21

3. Preschool children   40

4. Schoolchildren   47

5. Elderly people   58

Section 2: Social Aspects of Nutrition

6. Religious restrictions and cultural beliefs   71

7. Vegetarianism and food beliefs   75

8. Low income families   81

9. Nutrition and sport   92

Section 3: The Prevention of Ill Health

10. Coronary heart disease   99

11. Osteoporosis   125

12. Weight management   134

13. Dental health   146

14. Food hygiene   151

Appendices

1. The Balance of Good Health   159

2. Hygiene rules for the kitchen   161

RCGP Quality Network
Nutrition in General Practice Working Party

Dr Colin Waine OBE, FRCGP, FRCPath
  (*Chairman*)
Director of Primary Care
Sunderland Health Commission

Professor WPT James MA, MD, DSc,
  FRCP, FRCP(Ed), FRSE
Director
Rowett Research Institute
Aberdeen

Dr Judith Buttriss PhD, SRD (*Editor*)
Senior Nutritionist
National Dairy Council
London

Dr Margaret Lawson PhD, SRD
Senior Lecturer in Paediatric Nutrition
Department of Child Health
Institute of Child Health
University of London

Ms Josephine Cotterell BSc, SRD
Nutritionist
National Dairy Council
London

Mrs Georgina Lonsdale BSc
Home Economist
Flour Advisory Bureau
London

Dr Colin Smith MSc, FRCGP
Assistant Regional Adviser (Audit) in
  General Practice
South East Thames Region

Acknowledgement

The Royal College of General Practitioners thanks the National Dairy Council for the substantial contribution it has made towards publication of the three parts of *Nutrition in General Practice*, of which this is the second.

Preface to Part 2

Developments in 1994

Since publication of Part 1 at the beginning of 1994, there have been several developments nationally which are likely to have an impact on the work of the primary health care team in relation to nutrition.

The Balance of Good Health

First, in July 1994, a guide to helping the public choose a healthier diet, called *The Balance of Good Health* (see Appendix 1), was launched under the auspices of the Health of the Nation's Nutrition Task Force. The purpose of the guide is to help people understand and enjoy healthy eating and the Department of Health hopes that doctors and health professionals will make use of it in their work.

The food groupings used in the guide are essentially the same as those discussed in Chapter 9 of Part 1 of *Basic Principles of Nutrition*, but in addition a fifth group is included — "fatty and sugary foods", which were described as occasional foods in Part 1.

Increasing prevalence of overweight/obesity

Since the publication of Part 1, statistics mentioned in the text have worsened, in particular those relating to overweight/obesity. We stated then that almost 50% of adults are overweight. In 1993, more than 50% of adults were overweight (Bennett et al., 1995). More men (57%) than women (48%) were overweight/obese and more women (16%) than men (13%) were obese.

Clearly more needs to be done if a reduction in the prevalance of obesity — a Health of the Nation target — is to be achieved.

Core Curriculum

Another development has been the launch in November 1994 of a core curriculum for teaching nutrition to doctors and professionals other than dietitians and nutritionists. Again produced under the auspices of the Health of the Nation's Nutrition Task Force, this document is called *Core Curriculum for Nutrition in the Education of Health Professionals*.

The aims of the document are to:

- outline the nutrition requirements for the Health of the Nation strategy
- specify the aims of nutrition education and training for health professionals
- describe the current situation for education and training in nutrition
- provide guidance on developing the nutritional components of training.

The *Core Curriculum* considers the need for nutrition education and training during three periods of professional life:

- basic education and training, leading to the acquisition of a basic professional qualification
- post-basic education and training — formal education and training which are undertaken after basic training, and which result in the acquisition of a further, possibly specialist, qualification
- continuing education — formal or informal education, which is an important part of professional development and fitness to practise.

The document identifies a series of learning outcomes considered necessary to enable practice team members to modify public opinion about nutrition and to encourage adherence to dietary change. These are to:

- appreciate the importance and relevance of nutrition to the promotion of good health, the prevention and treatment of disease
- describe the basic scientific principles of human nutrition
- identify nutrition-related problems in individuals and in the community
- give consistent and sound dietary advice to people in an appropriate manner and know when and how to refer to a state registered dietitian for more specific advice
- know and be able to promote and explain current dietary recommendations and the advantages of breast feeding
- provide appropriate and safe clinical nutritional support, or know when and how to refer to a state registered dietitian or other specialist in clinical nutrition
- understand the relative costs and benefits of nutritional compared with other approaches to preventive and therapeutic care
- assess the validity of nutritional literature and nutritional reports in the media.

The range of topics, an understanding of which is believed to be necessary to achieve these outcomes, is split in the core curriculum into three areas, which are similar to those adopted in the RCGP's series of three publications produced under the general title *Nutrition in General Practice*:

- Principles of nutritional science
- Public health nutrition
- Clinical nutrition and nutritional support.

It is believed that the College's series of publications on nutrition will be of major importance in the context of the new core curriculum.

Reference

Bennett N et al. (1995) *Health Survey for England 1993*. Office of Population Censuses and Surveys. London, HMSO.

Preface to Part 1

THERE may be general practitioners who doubt the importance and value of good nutrition in maintaining well-being, but if so, they must be unaware that nutrition, the process by which food is eaten and utilized by the body, is fundamental to the maintenance of activity and growth, to the maintenance of health, and to the prevention and management of many common diseases and syndromes. Without the energy and nutrients derived from our food, growth and activity could not occur. Also, dietary imbalances are prominent features of many clinical syndromes. Adequate and appropriate nutrition is therefore essential to life.

Yet, surprisingly, nutrition does not figure prominently in the undergraduate medical curriculum and appears hardly at all in vocational training for general practice.

The problem

Such is the ease with which nutrition usually occurs that it is all too often taken for granted and it is only when it is disturbed that it becomes of clinical interest. Yet, the reality is that almost half the adults in Britain are overweight. Recent data show that the proportion of the population that is overweight has been increasing steadily in recent years: the 1991 Health Survey for England indicates that 45% of adult women are overweight (including 16% who are obese) and 53% of men are overweight (including 13% who are obese) (OPCS, 1993).

Furthermore, 69% of men and 70% of women have cholesterol concentrations above the desirable average for total serum cholesterol, with concentrations remaining at 5.8 mmol/litre in men and 5.9 mmol/litre in women.

Findings are little better for the other major risk factors for coronary heart disease. Only 12% of men and 11% of women are free from the four major risk factors: smoking, raised blood pressure, raised cholesterol and lack of physical activity.

A large number of diseases common in affluent societies have a nutritional basis which interacts with other factors such as genetics, smoking, and lack of exercise. For example, coronary heart disease, diabetes, diverticular disease of the colon, gallstones and dental caries all have associations with the Western diet with its relative excess of saturates and deficiency of fibre-rich, starchy foods.

The need

In Britain, fat provides about 42% of food energy, carbohydrate 45%, and protein the remaining 13%. These proportions need to be modified so that fat provides, on average, no more than 35% of energy intake with the balance being made up by an increased consumption of starchy, fibre-rich carbohydrates.

Given the importance of diet in the management of such common conditions as coronary heart disease, diabetes and obesity, the lack of training in nutrition for doctors and nurses is a significant omission. In spite of general practitioners' scant knowledge of nutrition and because diet is viewed as being so important in public health terms, the government has set a national agenda on nutrition which is described in the white paper, *The Health of the Nation* (Secretary of State for Health, 1992). The Health of the Nation initiative has set a series of targets, four of which are about nutrition, and members of the primary health care team are ideally placed in the front line of the health service to help in achieving the improvements in morbidity and mortality which are essential to securing a healthier nation (RCGP, 1987). However, it is important that general practitioners and other professionals should have the knowledge and information on which to base relevant and practical advice.

The Royal College of General Practitioners, recognizing this need well in advance of the publication of *The Health of the Nation*, set up a working party charged with the production of a manual on nutrition for primary care workers.

Aims

The manual has been prepared to help general practitioners, practice nurses and other primary health care professionals to give scientifically based and practical dietary advice to their practice population.

More specifically, the aims are:

1. To demonstrate to general practitioners and primary care teams aspects of the British diet that are at variance with current nutrition guidelines and targets, and show how these can contribute to ill health and disease.

2. To provide them with a clear understanding of the current knowledge of the mechanisms by which poor nutrition brings about ill health.

3. To provide them with information and methods to apply this understanding to the needs of individual patients and to the community as a whole.

4. To encourage them to try to bring about and monitor beneficial change for patients in general.

Contents

The manual will appear in three parts. The first part deals with the basic principles of nutrition, the second will deal with the role of nutrition in the promotion of health and prevention of disease, and the third with nutrition in the management of existing disease.

1. *Basic Principles of Nutrition*

This first part begins by considering nutrition in the context of the Health of the Nation targets and then goes on to discuss the broader government guidelines on nutrition — the dietary reference values — and their practical implementation. Practical suggestions are given regarding planning and implementing a nutrition policy at local level and on assessing and advising on diet.

2. *Promoting Health and Preventing Disease*

In the second part, the social aspects of nutrition are explored, as it is essential to understand these if changes in lifestyle relating to eating habits are to be achieved. Topics include vegetarianism and religious restrictions which influence food choice. The differing needs of different age groups are also considered, for example pre-conception, pregnancy and breast feeding; infants, schoolchildren and adolescents; and elderly people.

Particular attention is given to dental caries, overweight and obesity, the prevention of osteoporosis, and coronary heart disease.

3. *Nutrition in the Management of Disease*

In the third part, nutritional issues relating to the management of specific diseases are explored, for example anaemia in children and in women, liver and renal diseases, diabetes mellitus, as well as conditions such as malabsorption, food intolerance and allergy.

In addition, consideration is given to conditions requiring nutritional support (for example HIV infection, terminal illness), psychosocial aspects of nutrition (eating disorders), and alcohol and drug dependency.

References

Office of Population Censuses and Surveys (1993) *Health Survey for England, 1991.* A Survey carried out by the Social Survey Division of OPCS on behalf of the Department of Health. London, HMSO.

Royal College of General Practitioners (1987) *The Front Line of the Health Service. Report from General Practice 25.* London, RCGP.

Secretary of State for Health (1992) *The Health of the Nation. A Strategy for Health in England.* Cm 1986. London, HMSO.

Section 1:
The Needs of Specific Age Groups

Preconception, pregnancy and lactation

Key points

Preconception

1. The health and nutritional status of women prior to conception and during the first trimester is important, because the fetus is most susceptible to environmental influences, including nutritional imbalance, in the early weeks of pregnancy.

2. New research has resulted in a totally different approach to supplementation with folic acid. A 0.4 mg daily supplement is advised for all women of childbearing age because of the importance of folate in early pregnancy. A larger supplement of 4 mg is advised for those women who have had a previous child with a neural tube defect; it is particularly important that this group of women should receive advice on folate intake.

3. Apart from folic acid, to avoid the need for supplementation during pregnancy and to help ensure women enter pregnancy well nourished, opportunities such as those presented at contraception advice clinics should be taken **prior to pregnancy** to ensure that women's general nutrition, but in particular intakes of iron, calcium and essential fatty acids are adequate. Imbalances in body weight should also be corrected prior to pregnancy where possible. This is a new approach to management.

4. Smoking and drinking alcohol excessively during pregnancy both present a risk to the health of the fetus, as well as that of the mother. The embryo is particularly vulnerable in the early weeks before pregnancy is confirmed.

Pregnancy and lactation

5. The need for some nutrients increases during pregnancy and still further during lactation.

6. The increase in requirement for energy in pregnancy is small in most women. However, during lactation there is a considerable increase in the mother's energy needs.

7. Pregnant women and those who might become pregnant should avoid liver and liver products such as pâté, as there is the possibility that they may contain large quantities of vitamin A.

8. Adequate attention to food hygiene is particularly important for pregnant women. In addition specific foods (for example, pâtés and soft cheeses) which have been linked with the bacteria *Listeria monocytogenes* should be avoided by pregnant women.

9. As a result of new knowledge, a number of changes in policy and practice can now be recommended. In particular, vulnerable groups of women can be identified who may benefit from specific nutrition advice and from opportunistic monitoring of factors such as weight gain, iron status and calcium intake, for example. This monitoring should not be restricted to the pregnancy itself.

For many years now there has been a general feeling that in affluent countries such as Britain, there should be little cause for concern about the influence of maternal nutritional status on the fetus. It is frequently stated that although good nutrition is important to pregnancy outcome, the fetus is protected against nutritional adversity by the mother and that it is she, not the fetus, who will suffer if nutritional status is poor. Although to some extent this may be true, recent developments in the area of prenatal nutrition have once again focused attention on this subject, both in relation to the immediate health of the fetus and longer term health in adulthood.

Preconception

The time immediately before conception, and during the first trimester, when cell differentiation is most rapid, is the most critical period for embryonic and fetal development. It is at this time that adverse environmental influences, notably maternal exposure to smoking, alcohol, certain drugs, and viral infections, are most likely to cause damage to the developing baby. There is evidence too that imbalances in maternal diet at this time may have adverse effects (Wharton, 1992) and it is now clear that women should have access to appropriate information on the importance of their diet **prior to conception** and in the early days of pregnancy, particularly as many women will be unaware that they have conceived during much of this vulnerable period. Such information should be available to girls as part of health education programmes in schools.

It is now clear that it is vital that women are encouraged to prepare for pregnancy by reducing their alcohol intake (see below), giving up smoking and consuming an adequate diet, especially with regard to folic acid (see below). As yet, this has not been fully appreciated by either doctors or the women they advise.

Opportunities such as presented at contraception advice clinics should be taken to emphasize the importance of good nutrition. The services of the dietitian can be used to provide detailed advice for those women whose diets are particularly poor. Other opportunities may arise through consultations associated with smear tests and routine health checks.

Much remains unknown about the precise influence of maternal nutrition on fetal development, but certain areas can be highlighted as being of particular importance.

Body weight

Problems of both underweight and overweight are best corrected before conception because manipulation of body weight during pregnancy may be a threat to the fetus.

Underweight (low weight for height) is generally assumed to be indicative of marginal tissue reserves of nutrients. Undernutrition is certainly associated with a fall in the ability to conceive, as is seen in famine. For example, in the Dutch famine of 1944/5 amenorrhoea was common and there was evidence that the sudden fall in energy intake inhibited ovulation (Campbell, 1991). Certainly there was a fall in birth rate. Women who were pregnant during the Dutch famine delivered infants with reduced birthweights, placental weights, length at birth and head circumference, mainly attributable to the effects of famine in the third trimester, although perinatal mortality was not affected.

Overweight mothers have a slightly increased risk of late pregnancy complications, including hypertensive disease, gestational diabetes, prolonged labour and increased perinatal mortality.

The subject of optimal weight gain during pregnancy has been considered in detail by a subcommittee of the Institute of Medicine of the US National Academy of Sciences (1990) and is discussed in more detail on pages 8–10.

Intake of specific nutrients

There is evidence from animal studies that both nutrient deficiencies and excesses occurring during embryogenesis (the first two months of gestation) may result in fetal malformations; however, information relating to human pregnancies is much more limited. Two specific nutrients should be highlighted.

Vitamin A

Congenital abnormalities of the eyes, brain and skeleton have resulted from the administration of very high doses of vitamin A to experimental animals. Although the precise dose-response relationship is uncertain in humans, there is also some evidence that high intakes in humans are teratogenic (cause congenital malformations) and it is suggested that excessive intakes would be those above 3300 µg per day (DH, 1991). Thus, in the UK, women who are, or who might become pregnant are advised not to take supplements containing vitamin A unless specifically recommended to do so by their doctor or antenatal clinic (CMO, 1990). Additionally, because of the finding of exceptionally high amounts of the vitamin in types of liver commonly consumed in Britain (13 000–40 000 µg/100 g), pregnant women and those who might become pregnant are also advised not to eat liver or its products, for example pâté, for the time being (CMO, 1990). Nevertheless, such women still require vitamin A (see Part 1, Appendix 1 for dietary reference values) and so they should be advised to consume more of the foods which contain the precursor of vitamin A, beta-carotene (yellow/orange and green pigmented vegetables and fruits).

Folate

The report of an Expert Advisory Group (DH, 1992a) recommends that **to prevent recurrence of neural tube defects (NTD)**, women with a history of a previous child with neural tube defects should take a daily supplement of 5 mg of folic acid if they are trying to conceive or are at risk of becoming pregnant (a 4 mg dose is not yet available as a licensed product). They should continue this supplement until week 12 of the pregnancy. This recommendation is based on results of a large randomized trial (MRC Vitamin Study Research Group, 1991) in which there was a significant reduction in recurrence of neural tube defects in women who received a daily supplement of 4 mg

folic acid (reference nutrient intake, 0.2 mg per day) prior to their pregnancy and during the early weeks.

To prevent the first occurrence of neural tube defects a smaller daily folic acid supplement of 0.4 mg (400 µg) is recommended for all women of childbearing age. This supplement should also be continued to week 12 of pregnancy.

In addition, it is recommended that all women of childbearing age:

- eat more folate-rich foods (Table 1.1)
- eat foods fortified with folic acid (for example, fortified breakfast cereals and fortified bread).

In the context of neural tube defects, this supplement is thought to be needed only in the weeks immediately prior to conception and during the first 12 weeks. However, the advice is directed to **all** women of childbearing age, as a large proportion of pregnancies are unplanned. It is also thought that only some subgroups of the female population are susceptible to NTD births, but as yet these subgroups cannot be identified. Hence the advice should be given to all women of childbearing age.

Women who have not been taking a supplement and find they are pregnant should begin to take daily 0.4 mg supplements at the earliest opportunity and continue these until week 12 of their pregnancy.

This advice on the need for extra folate supersedes that in the report on dietary reference values (DH, 1991) in which a reference nutrient intake (RNI) of 0.2 mg (200 µg) was advised for women in general, and 0.3 mg in pregnancy. (Current intakes are typically about 0.2 mg per day.) For further discussion of this issue see Part 1, page 15.

It may seem strange that, for the first time, folate pills are being advised in this way. However, the public health burden of neural tube defects is considered sufficiently great for this advice to be necessary, particularly

Table 1.1 *Food sources of folate/folic acid*

Rich sources (more than 100 μg [0.1 mg] per serving*)
Fresh, raw, or cooked** Brussels sprouts, asparagus, spinach, kale, cooked black eye beans
Breakfast cereals (if fortified with folic acid)
Soft grain bread (if fortified with folic acid)

Good sources (50–100 μg [0.05–0.1 mg] per serving*)
Fresh, raw, frozen and cooked** broccoli, spring greens, cabbage, green beans, cauliflower, peas, beansprouts, okra, cooked soya beans, iceberg lettuce, parsnips, chick peas. (Larger 150–200 g) portions of broccoli, cauliflower and spring greens will supply more than 100 μg)
Kidneys, yeast and beef extracts

Moderate sources (15–50 μg [0.015–0.05 mg] per serving)
Potatoes, most other fresh and cooked vegetables, most fruits, most nuts, tahini
Bread (100 g), brown rice, wholegrain pasta, oats, Weetaflakes, Weetabix
Cheese, yogurt, milk (pint), eggs, salmon, beef, game

Poor sources (less than 15 μg [less than 0.015 mg] per serving)
White rice, white pasta, soft drinks, sugar, most pastries, cakes, most other meat and fish
Most other breakfast cereals (not fortified with folic acid)

Inhibitors*
Alcoholic drinks

*Minimum recommended portion sizes are 100 g of these vegetables.
**Based on vegetables boiled for 10 to 20 minutes. Steamed, stir-fried and microwaved vegetables cooked for a shorter time will lose less.
***Inhibits folate absorption.

Source: Adapted from Department of Health (1992a).

for those women who choose to eat few foods rich in folate. It is possible to obtain sufficient folate from food but careful food choices would need to be made and large quantities of folate-rich foods would be needed daily (Table 1.1).

Note that liver is not included in Table 1.1. It is an excellent source of folate but for the time being should not be consumed by pregnant women because of the possibility of a high vitamin A content.

It is also important to note that absorption and utilization of folate is inhibited by alcohol, for example a glass of wine with a meal.

Other nutrients

As far as other vitamins and minerals are concerned, there is little information available about their influence on the development of the embryo or the fetus.

However, it is obviously important to optimize the body's stores of nutrients before conception so as to enter pregnancy well nourished. This is best achieved by consuming a varied diet, based on nutrient-rich foods, which meets energy requirements (see Appendix 1 and Part 1, page 31). Diet prior to pregnancy and between pregnancies can be as important as diet during pregnancy.

Reference nutrient intakes for **calcium** and **iron** do not increase for pregnancy, although requirements rise to meet the needs of fetus and placenta. It is assumed that stores are adequate to cope with pregnancy and that these stores are mobilized (see pages 13–14). It is therefore worth paying particular attention to intakes of these nutrients in women considering pregnancy. This can be tackled opportunistically and via clinics attended by women of childbearing age.

Poor iron status is common among young women (see page 13). About 34% of British women have low iron stores (OPCS, 1993) and this rises to 47% in women under 45 years. Ideally poor iron status should be tackled prior to pregnancy because anaemia in the mother is associated with a high placental to birthweight ratio, which carries implications for health in adulthood (Barker, 1992). (See also page 11 and Chapter 10, page 118.) In this respect, a change in practice is required: efforts should be made to identify women with low iron stores prior to pregnancy, by testing serum ferritin levels. Currently about 15% to 30% of women have no stores of iron at the time they become pregnant.

Brain development is rapid during the latter part of fetal life and during the first two years of life. Important materials for this process are the essential fatty acids and their long chain metabolites (see page 15). Consequently, it has been suggested that maternal intake of **essential fatty acids** is particularly crucial. These are found in a range of foods in small amounts, but requirements can readily be met by consuming oil-rich fish such as mackerei, salmon, herring, sardines or pilchards twice weekly (BNF, 1992), by eating plenty of green, leafy vegetables, and by eating small amounts of a pure vegetable oil, for example in salad dressing.

Alcohol

Women considering pregnancy should avoid alcoholic drinks or reduce intake to a minimum.

Although there is no clear association between moderate drinking (50–100 g of alcohol [5–10 units] per week) and effects on the fetus (Wright et al., 1983; Beattie, 1992), there are no clear data on which to base a safe lower limit. It would seem that 10 g (1 unit) per day is unlikely to be harmful. However in the absence of clear evidence, women are best advised to avoid alcohol completely before

conception and during pregnancy (Royal College of Physicians, 1987). (See also section on folate, page 6.)

However, alcohol has long been recognized as a potential cause of fetal malformation (Beattie, 1992) and in 1973, Jones and colleagues proposed the term 'fetal alcohol syndrome' (FAS) to describe the various phenomena seen in infants born to women who had drunk excessively in pregnancy. The syndrome is characterized by a consistent pattern of congenital abnormalities of the cardiac system, skeleton, eyes and mouth. Mental retardation is also a feature of the syndrome. Fetal alcohol syndrome is associated with regular excessive drinking (more than 80 grams [8 units] of alcohol per day).

The fetus is not readily able to metabolize alcohol as the necessary liver enzyme systems are too immature, and the effects of moderate but regular drinking during pregnancy, for example of more than 100 g (10 units) of alcohol per week, may be more subtle and have not been properly defined. Women taking more than 10 drinks a week should be advised to reduce their intake and special counselling should be available for those unable to comply (Murray-Lyon, 1989). Particular attention should be paid to the folate intake of women unable to comply with advice to restrict alcohol consumption (see page 6).

Smoking

There is evidence that smoking may reduce the fertility of women (Wynn and Wynn, 1981) and increase the risk of spontaneous abortion and congenital abnormality (Himmelberger et al., 1978). Men who smoke have reduced testosterone levels (Briggs, 1973) and sperm counts (Hendry, 1979) and a higher frequency of morphologically abnormal sperm (Evans et al., 1981). Smoking is also known to reduce birthweight and to influence the health of the infant (Rantakallio, 1978). However a number of studies have suggested that the influence of smoking may be explained, at least in part, by differences in nutritional intake. Findings from the St George's Hospital birthweight study (Haste et al., 1991) indicated that intakes of micronutrients and fibre were lower in smokers at both 28 and 36 weeks and that, in late pregnancy, smokers reduced their intakes more than non-smokers. Low intakes of protein, zinc, riboflavin and thiamin at 36 weeks and a fall in intakes of these nutrients and of iron between 28 and 36 weeks seemed to affect birthweight; in other words, low intakes were associated with lower birthweights.

In particular, smoking is thought to increase vitamin C requirements because the vitamin, a potent antioxidant, is used to counteract and process the damaging free radicals and toxic compound in cigarette smoke.

Women who do not smoke are less likely to have a small-for-dates baby. Smoking is thought to have this effect by decreasing uterine blood flow and hence the quantities of nutrients reaching the fetus. Low birthweight carries the greatest probability of death, morbidity and brain damage. It can carry with it a degree of mental handicap which persists after the neonatal stage (see page 11).

Work by Barker's group has indicated that low birthweight coupled with a high placental weight predicts a variety of adverse conditions in adulthood, including coronary heart disease itself and related factors such as high blood pressure (Barker, 1992). In addition, Golding and colleagues (1990) have suggested that the offspring of women who smoke have a greater chance of developing cancer during childhood.

There is no doubt that women should be strongly discouraged from smoking before and during pregnancy, although campaigns directed at stopping smoking should take into account the complex reasons why people choose to smoke. If women are unable to comply with advice to stop smoking, particular attention should be paid to their nutrient intake, especially that of vitamin C, in order partially to counteract the effect of smoking on the fetus. Smokers probably need up to three times the quantity of vitamin C required daily by non-smokers in order to maintain the same circulating and tissue levels of the vitamin (DH, 1991).

Caffeine

Although it has been suggested that there may be associations between consumption of caffeinated beverages and reduced fertility and defects in fetal development, these effects have not been substantiated. Although women who may become pregnant should not consume excessive amounts of these drinks, a moderate intake, for example four or five cups of tea or coffee a day, is unlikely to be harmful. Cola drinks also contain caffeine.

Action points for those advising women considering pregnancy

- Record body mass index (BMI) and advise on weight gain/loss, as necessary
- Counsel those who smoke or who drink excessively (more than 14 units a week)
- Determine red cell folate
- Determine serum ferritin
- Provide advice on folic acid supplements and folate intake in general
- Discuss intake of essential fatty acids, especially n-3 fatty acids (oil-rich fish).

Pregnancy

As indicated in Table 1.2, the processes of pregnancy and lactation influence both the nutrient and energy requirements of the mother. However, there is a considerable amount of maternal adaptation, so that the requirements for many nutrients and for energy in the early stages of pregnancy are not increased. Thus the idea of 'eating for two' is definitely a myth. However, the quality of the diet remains very important.

Energy requirements and weight gain

Contrary to popular belief, for most women in Western societies such as the UK, the

Table 1.2 *Increments in the estimated average requirements for energy and reference nutrient intakes for pregnant and lactating women*

	Non-pregnant (age 19–50)	Pregnant	Lactating 0–4 months	Lactating after 4 months
Energy, kcal	1940	+200*	+450–570	+480**
Protein, g	45.0	+6	+11	+8
Thiamin, mg	0.8	+0.1*	+0.2	+0.2
Riboflavin, mg	1.1	+0.3	+0.5	+0.5
Niacin, mg	13.0	—	+2	+2
Vitamin B_{12}, µg	1.5	—	+0.5	+0.5
Folate, µg	200	+100***	+60	+60
Vitamin C, mg	40	+10	+30	+30
Vitamin A, µg	600	+100	+350	+350
Vitamin D, µg	—	10	10	10
Calcium, mg	700	—	+550	+550
Phosphorus, mg	550	—	+440	+440
Magnesium, mg	270	—	+50	+50
Zinc, mg	7.0	—	+6.0	+2.5
Copper, mg	1.2	—	+0.3	+0.3
Selenium, µg	60	—	+15	+15
Iron, mg	14.8	—	—	—

*Last trimester only.

**Assuming weaning is begun at 3–4 months, if breast milk is the sole source of nourishment, on average an extra 90 kcal/day would be needed.

***This recommendation was published prior to concerns about folate intake in early pregnancy. Until the twelfth week, women are now advised to take a 0.4 mg (400 µg) supplement, in addition to their normal dietary intake (typically about 0.2 mg).

See Part 1, Appendix 1 for reference nutrient intakes for non-pregnant women under the age of 19.

Source: Department of Health (1991).

additional energy requirements imposed by pregnancy are quite small (DH, 1991).

However, this energy cost does not appear to be matched by a comparable increase in appetite, and surveys have shown an average increase in energy intake of only 100 kcal per day, and this is seen in the third trimester only (DH, 1991). The disparity between the calculated values and experimental findings may be explained by an adaptation in basal metabolic rate and reduction in physical activity, but more experimental evidence is needed. Because of the disparity and lack of confirming evidence, the estimated average requirement (EAR) was set, cautiously, at an extra 200 kcal per day in the third trimester. But it was recognized that women who enter pregnancy underweight for height or who do

not, like the majority of women, reduce their activity levels, may need more (DH, 1991). Similarly, some women will require no increment in energy intake because they reduce physical activity levels substantially.

In the UK, average weight gain in pregnancy is 12.5 kg. The question of appropriate or desirable weight gain in pregnancy was addressed by a subcommittee of the Institute of Medicine of the US National Academy of Sciences (1990). The subcommittee concluded that pre-pregnancy weight for height is the most important determinant of gestational weight gain and that women overweight at conception gain less weight than do thinner women. However, a wide variation in weight gain for women with normal pregnancy outcomes (birthweights 3 to 4 kg; 39 to 41 weeks' gestation) was observed for women in different weight for height ranges. The subcommittee noted that there was a large body of evidence indicating that gestational weight gain, particularly in the second and third trimesters, was an important determinant of fetal growth. Low gestational weight gain is associated with an increased risk of fetal growth retardation, which in turn has adverse effects on subsequent growth and possibly on neuro-behavioural development, and on infant mortality (see section on Smoking).

The following ranges of weight gain were recommended for pregnant women by the subcommittee:

Pre-pregnancy body mass index (BMI)	Recommended total gain (kg)
19.8 (underweight)	12.5–18.0
19.8–26.0 (normal weight)	11.5–16.0
26.0–29.0 (overweight)	7.0–11.5

These figures are somewhat higher than those proposed previously. The increase in the recommended range for women of normal weight was based on the reduced risk of giving birth to an infant with intrauterine growth retardation when weight gain was slightly higher.

Weight gain in pregnancy

Regular monitoring of the weight of pregnant women is still advised. However, there is little evidence to show that routine weighing during pregnancy is able to assess accurately or influence fetal growth, and can in some women cause anxiety (Dawes et al., 1992). Weight gain over the whole pregnancy, rather than monthly gain, is of greater predictive value for low birth weight.

For women with a normal pre-pregnancy body mass index, the subcommittee recommended a target weight gain at a rate of 0.4 kg (approximately 1 lb) per week during the second and third trimesters of pregnancy.

For underweight women a weight gain of 0.5 kg/week is recommended.

Dietary advice will be needed by women with a low pre-pregnancy body mass index or who fail to gain weight at an appropriate rate. If such women have been physically very active, they may need to consider reducing their exercise routine. Such women sometimes eat quite small amounts of food and so energy intake may need to be increased by substitutions, for example whole milk for skimmed milk, during the periods of pregnancy and lactation.

For overweight women a weight gain of 0.3 kg/week is recommended.

Average weight gains of more than 0.5 kg/week should be considered too fast and action should be taken (ensure that the scales being used are accurate). Blood pressure has been shown to be higher in those with the greatest weight gain. Although excess weight gain is not diagnostic of pre-eclampsia, it should alert general practitioners to monitor women for other signs and symptoms of pre-eclampsia, which has been associated with premature delivery (Dimperio et al., 1992).

For women in whom weight gain is judged to be too fast, guidance should be given on reducing fat intake, compensating for the reduction in calories by an increase in starchy carbohydrate foods. As such foods are filling, it is likely that overall energy intake will fall slightly and slow down weight gain.

Very high gestational weight gain is associated with high birthweight and this in turn leads to high risks of forceps or caesarean deliveries, birth trauma, asphyxia and mortality. However, unless there is a real risk of complications, severe restriction of energy intake in pregnancy should be avoided because of the risk of associated fetal growth retardation. Therefore obesity in the mother is best corrected before or after the pregnancy (Campbell, 1983).

Nutrient intake

Low birthweight is associated with high rates of still births and neonatal and infant mortality. Furthermore, the work of Barker and colleagues (1992) has shown that low birthweight is associated with a higher incidence of chronic disorders, including cardiovascular disease in later life.

This serves to underline the importance of women entering pregnancy well nourished, and of good nutrition and adequate maternal weight gain during pregnancy. According to Barker's hypothesis, together these should help minimize the occurrence of low birth weight and hence the risk of chronic diseases such as coronary heart disease and associated risk factors, such as high blood cholesterol, hypertension and diabetes in middle age (Barker et al., 1993).

In the UK, birthweight is significantly related to both region and socio-economic group (OPCS, 1992). Socio-economic group encompasses many confounding variables, for example mothers from socio-economic groups 4 and 5 and Manual 3 tend to be younger, lighter and shorter and to smoke more. However, there is also evidence of differences in nutrient intake which may be important.

In a series of studies in women of low socio-economic status carried out in Hackney (Doyle et al., 1982; Crawford et al., 1986; Doyle et al., 1989; Wynn et al., 1994), mothers of babies with low birthweights (less than 2500 g) had lower intakes of nutrients, particularly micronutrients including the B vitamins, vitamin C, magnesium, folate and zinc, than mothers of normal weight infants.

The association between nutrient intake and birthweight appeared to be strongest in the first trimester of pregnancy. This research group was able to show a pronounced social class gradient in nutrient intake for several micronutrients and the pattern has also been observed in other data collected from pregnant mothers in London and Edinburgh (Schofield et al., 1989).

The fact that the association between nutrient intake in the second and third trimesters and birthweight is less pronounced emphasizes the importance of preconceptional nutrition and nutrition in early pregnancy — not just in relation to the early months of infancy but, according to Barker (1992), for health in adulthood too.

However, there remain a great many unanswered questions in this field, which will only be clarified as a result of further research. For example, perhaps other pregnancy end-points such as the subsequent potential of the mother to breast feed, the development of the infant's immune system and consequent reduced susceptibility to infection, and the time taken to reach particular development milestones may be influenced by nutrition later in pregnancy. These or others could eventually be seen as additional markers of successful pregnancy outcome in addition to birthweight.

Specific vitamins and minerals

Table 1.2 shows that the requirement for some nutrients increases in proportionally greater amounts than requirements for energy. It is accepted that maternal adaptation occurs and may protect the fetus against deficiency. However, the mother will obviously suffer in the long term at the expense of the fetus, if her own demands for nutrients cannot be met.

Calcium

Calcium requirements increase in pregnancy, particularly in the third trimester when calcification of the fetal skeleton occurs. But it is believed that these additional requirements can be met both by mobilization of maternal bone stores and by the increased efficiency of absorption of calcium. Hence no specific increment in calcium intake is recommended in pregnancy (DH, 1991). The exception to this is pregnant women under 18 years of age. In this case, there will be an exceptionally high demand for calcium to sustain the continued growth of the mother as well as of the fetus. Intakes of at least 800 mg per day are advised (1350 mg/day during breast feeding), especially if previous intake was poor.

Table 1.3 *Portions of foods which each contain about 230 mg calcium*

Dairy products
$^1/_3$ pint/190 ml semi-skimmed milk (or skimmed/whole)
1 oz/28 g Cheddar cheese (traditional or low fat)
1 pot yogurt (5 oz/140 g)
3 small pots fromage frais (11 oz/300 g)
$12^1/_2$ oz/ 350 g plain cottage cheese

Fish
2 canned sardines with bones (2 oz/56 g)
6 oz/ 168 g prawns
1 oz/28 g cooked whitebait
3 oz/84 g canned pilchards with bones
9 oz/250 g canned salmon (backbone removed)

Seeds and nuts
14 teaspoons sesame seeds ($1^1/_2$ oz/42 g)
2 packets sunflower seeds (7 oz/200 g)
4 oz/112 g almonds
6 oz/168 g hazelnuts

Bread and cereals
8 medium slices white or brown bread ($8^1/_2$ oz/240 g)
4 currant buns ($8^1/_2$ oz/240 g)
16 medium slices wholemeal bread (1 lb 1 oz/480 g)
3 white pitta bread (9 oz/250 g)

Fruit
6 dried figs (3 oz/84 g)
12 oz/336 g dried apricots
4 oranges (1 lb 1 oz/480 g)

Vegetables
4 bunches watercress (5 oz/ 140 g)
12 oz/336 g cooked spring greens, 1 lb 8 oz/672 g before preparation
1 lb 4 oz/560 g broccoli
7 oz/196 g okra
6 oz/168 g boiled curly kale
1 lb 7 oz/650 g green beans

Beans and soya products
1 large can red kidney beans or baked beans (15 oz/420 g)
$1^1/_2$ oz/42 g steamed tofu
$^1/_3$–$^1/_2$ pint (approx)/190–290 ml fortified soya milk (calcium content
  varies from product to product)

It should also be emphasized that in keeping the calcium reference nutrient intake at pre-pregnancy levels, it is assumed that the mother enters pregnancy well nourished and with adequate nutrient stores. Women who have had poor diets before becoming pregnant will need to ensure that they consume adequate amounts of calcium-rich foods (Table 1.3) if they are not to endanger their own future bone health by drawing too heavily upon the calcium stored in their own skeleton.

Women whose pregnancy has produced more than one baby and those who have had closely spaced pregnancies may experience considerable depletion of their calcium stores.

Such women may benefit from particular advice on calcium intake post-pregnancy, for example daily consumption of at least half a pint of semi-skimmed milk, or more if they are breast feeding.

Certain women, such as Asian and Chinese women and those following a vegan diet, may experience specific problems in achieving an adequate calcium intake and this should be addressed, particularly if it is accompanied by poor vitamin D status. Ideally needs should be met from food, but on occasions supplements may be necessary. In addition, Asian women are likely to start their pregnancy with a low body weight, which carries implications for the pregnancy outcome (see page 10).

Although there may be some adaptation of calcium metabolism in lactation, it is currently assumed that quite a large increment in dietary calcium intake is needed to meet requirements of mother and child (DH, 1991). A normal output of breast milk provides the baby with about 300 mg of calcium per day.

Mothers may need particular advice on meeting these high intakes. Milk and its products (cheese and yogurt) are rich and particularly bioavailable sources of calcium. Skimmed, semi-skimmed and whole milk contain similar amounts of calcium (about 700 mg per pint) and 50 grams (about 2 oz) of hard cheese (full or reduced fat) plus 1 small pot of yogurt will together supply the same amount. Table 1.3 shows portions of foods which each contain about 230 mg calcium (the amount in a glass of milk). In some cases the portions shown are quite large to emphasize that though these foods contain calcium, they need to be eaten in large amounts. These portions take no account of bioavailability; in other words, portion for portion calcium will generally be better absorbed from milk group foods than from vegetables.

Iron
More iron is required in pregnancy, mainly to supply the growing fetus, the placenta and to increase the maternal red cell mass. Pregnant women are therefore at greater risk of iron deficiency anaemia because of inadequate iron intake. Provided a woman has adequate iron stores on entering pregnancy, additional requirements can be met without further increase in intake because of mobilization of these stores, cessation of menstruation and increased intestinal absorption of dietary iron.

The problem is that many women do not have adequate stores of iron and these women may require supplementation, especially if their dietary intake of iron remains low. There is a view that the proportion of iron absorbed is improved when supplements are given intermittently, for example every few days, rather than daily (see Part 3, Anaemia in Adults and Children).

Ideally poor iron status should be tackled before pregnancy begins (see page 7). Women at particular risk of low iron stores are:

- those who have had a number of babies, particularly when the pregnancies have been closely spaced
- those on a vegan or vegetarian diet
- those in lower socio-economic groups if diet is poor or restricted
- those in whom blood loss during menstruation is typically heavy.

Iron depletion is generally described in three stages of increasing severity (Bothwell et al., 1979):

1. depletion of iron stores
2. impaired haemoglobin production
3. iron deficiency anaemia.

It is believed that the first stage is in fact very common in British women (see page 7) and its existence can be established by measurement of serum ferritin levels, a measure of iron stores.

There has been and continues to be much debate about whether women should or should not routinely be supplemented with iron in pregnancy. The situation is further complicated by the physiological changes and adaptations occurring during pregnancy, such as haemodilution (expansion of the blood volume), which can lead to mis-interpretation of the normal laboratory indices of iron status in pregnancy (Lind, 1983).

Unnecessary administration of iron carries disadvantages, including gastro-intestinal disturbance and competition with other minerals, such as zinc, for intestinal absorption. A more cost-effective and safe approach is the identification and supplementation of women displaying evidence of iron in-sufficiency (Lind, 1983). Such women should ideally be identified prior to conception (see page 7), before the physiological changes of pregnancy occur, but if necessary they can also be identified as a result of full blood counts undertaken periodically throughout pregnancy. There should be flexibility in the timing of these periodic checks but suitable times would be: at booking, 28 weeks, 36 weeks and after delivery. Follow-up is very important, particularly in those who are not regular attenders — failure to act because results are returned between appointments should be avoided.

Particular attention should be paid to opportunistic screening of at-risk women and targeting of advice for such groups.

Guidelines on expected iron levels for women are:

- **Non-pregnant women:**
  haemoglobin of 12 g/dl or above
  serum ferritin of 12 µg/dl or above
- **Pregnant women:**
  haemoglobin of 11 g/dl or above
  serum ferritin of 12 µg/dl or above

(See also Part 3, Anaemia in Children and Adults.)

For women first tested late in pregnancy, haemoglobin levels below 10 g/dl, in association with a mean cell volume (MCV) of 82 fl or less, or a progressive fall in MCV, indicate the need for dietary intervention and/or supplementation.

The most available sources of iron are offal, such as liver, and meat but pregnant women are now advised to avoid liver because of the discovery that it may contain high vitamin A levels (see page 5). Iron is present in cereals, vegetables, pulses and eggs, but it is less well absorbed from these foods. Meat, particularly red meat, is therefore a very important part of the diet of pregnant women. Vitamin C (in vegetables and fruits) enhances the absorption of iron and such foods should be eaten at the same meal as non-meat sources of iron (see Part 1 pages 16 and 29, and Appendix 2). Vitamin C may also help absorption of the iron in iron tablets. Tannins in teas inhibit the absorption of non-haem iron and so tea should not be drunk with non-meat meals containing iron. This is particularly important advice for vegetarians.

Women who follow a vegetarian diet are likely to have poorer iron intakes but adaptation to these intakes seems to enable a large proportion of them to maintain an adequate iron status. However, those who have recently adopted such an eating pattern ('new' vegetarians) may be more at risk.

Zinc
Zinc is involved in the processes of cell differentiation and replication and there is evidence of an increased need for zinc in pregnancy (DH, 1991). The consequences of mild zinc deficiency in human pregnancy are not as yet well defined. Although there have been suggestions that it may lead to con-genital malformation and intra-uterine growth retardation as well as complications, there is a lack of consistency in the findings of different studies (Hambidge, 1989). For the majority of healthy women it is considered probable that metabolic adapt-ation ensures adequate transfer of zinc to the fetus (DH, 1991), but further data on the prevalence of zinc deficiency and its effects are needed.

In lactation, it is believed that extra zinc is needed (DH, 1991). Red meat, wholegrain cereals, milk, cheese and nuts are good dietary sources.

Folic acid

As discussed on page 5 and in Part 1 (page 15), folic acid is an important nutrient in pregnancy and requirements increase in both pregnancy and lactation. Foods rich in folic acid include leafy green vegetables, legumes such as peas, potatoes, oranges, bananas, wholegrain cereals (some breakfast cereals are fortified with folate) (Table 1.1). Bovril and Marmite are also good sources but should only be consumed in small amounts because of their high sodium content.

Vitamin D

Vitamin D is important for the increased absorption and utilization of calcium during pregnancy. The levels of the active metabolite of vitamin D, 1,25-dihydroxycholecalciferol, are elevated in pregnancy (Paulson and Deluca, 1986) but the extent to which the increase is influenced by hormones, including prolactin, is uncertain.

The action of ultra violet light on the skin is the main source of vitamin D but good dietary sources include oily fish, eggs and fortified foods, such as margarine, some yogurts and some breakfast cereals.

Neonatal hypocalcaemia and dental enamel hypoplasia have been reported in infants born to mothers with poor vitamin D status (Cockburn et al., 1980). It is recommended that both pregnant and lactating women in the UK should receive supplementary vitamin D to achieve an intake of 10 μg per day (DH, 1991). This may be particularly important in women who receive little exposure to sunlight, such as Asian mothers and those living in northern Britain.

Essential fatty acids

The essential fatty acids and their metabolites are the major constituents of the brain's structure. Phospholipids make up about a quarter of the solid matter of the brain and are an integral part of the vascular system on which the brain depends. Rapid brain growth and phospholipid incorporation occurs during fetal and early neonatal life. This means that the lipid content of the diet during pregnancy and early infancy may be especially important with regard to subsequent brain development.

Brain growth is associated with an increase in incorporation of long chain polyunsaturated fatty acids into the phospholipids in the cerebral cortex. Studies in animals have indicated that extreme modification of dietary intake of the essential fatty acids — linoleic acid (C18:2 n-6) and α-linolenic acid (C18:3 n-3) — leads to alteration in the polyunsaturated fatty acid composition of the developing brain. These two fatty acids are described as 'essential' because they cannot be made in the body. They are the precursors for the long chain polyunsaturates, arachidonic acid, eicosopentaenoic acid (EPA) and docosahexaenoic acid (DHA). These long chain polyunsaturates are found in breast milk and are now in some infant formulae.

It has been suggested that low birthweight infants fed synthetic milks may have difficulty in making the quantity and type of fatty acids needed by the brain for its development (Lucas et al., 1992). This makes it particularly important that the fetus is provided with these particular fatty acids during pregnancy.

The dietary sources of other nutrients needed in increased amounts during pregnancy and lactation can be found in Part 1, Appendix 2.

Potential at-risk groups

The following groups may require special attention and advice, particularly if several of the characteristics are combined:

- **Adolescent pregnancies:** Girls under the age of 18 who become pregnant have to contend with their own needs for growth as well as those of the developing baby. Particular care needs to be paid with respect to the girl's diet during pregnancy, but also after the baby is born (particularly if she breast feeds) to ensure that her own stores are replenished.

- **Vegetarians (particularly 'new' vegetarians):** In people who have recently turned to a vegetarian eating pattern, the adaptive processes which enable lower intakes of essential nutrients to be adequate have yet to be developed. In addition, some people, particularly teenagers, who are 'vegetarian' do not eat the balanced and healthy diet eaten by many long-term vegetarians.

- **Asian women:** Low birthweight infants are fairly common among Asian women. This will in part be determined by their small stature and low pre-pregnancy weight, but diet may also play a part. Intake of some nutrients may be low, particularly among those who are vegetarian.

Dietary solutions to problems

Nausea and vomiting (morning sickness) are common symptoms in early pregnancy. Traditional advice has been that small, frequent snacks rather than large meals can help to alleviate the nausea, and that morning sickness may be helped by a snack at bedtime, and a plain biscuit or piece of toast and a hot drink before getting up in the morning. This advice may be helpful, and in addition some women benefit from avoiding coffee and tea.

Indigestion and heartburn are also common and again, small frequent snacks often help alleviate symptoms, as do avoiding spicy and fatty foods, eating slowly and sticking to those foods which the woman normally finds easy to digest. A glass of water can also be helpful. Frequent use of antacids should be avoided as these can bind to iron, making it unavailable, or reduce its bio-availability by neutralizing stomach acid.

Constipation can be relieved by eating more high fibre foods (see Part 1, page 6) and drinking plenty of fluid (6–8 glasses per day). Regular exercise, such as a daily 20-minute brisk walk, can also help. Iron tablets can be a cause of constipation — another reason for correcting iron status **before** pregnancy.

Food cravings are unlikely to have any adverse effect on the mother's health provided that there is no drastic change in diet such as omitting an entire food group.

Adequate regard for **food hygiene** is particularly important in pregnancy (see Chapter 14 and Appendix 2). There are three infections which women should be especially careful to avoid: listeriosis, salmonellosis and toxoplasmosis. Advice concerning these infections, issued by the Department of Health (1992b), can be summarized as follows:

- **Listeriosis:** Although very few cases have been reported in the UK, pregnant women should avoid foods where high levels of *Listeria* bacteria have been found. This means avoiding all types of pâté and soft and blue-veined varieties of cheeses (there is no risk with other hard cheeses, cottage cheese, processed cheese or cheese spread — the bacteria cannot survive). Any ready-prepared foods should not be eaten cold, and should be heated until they are piping hot. Also, fruit and vegetables should be washed well, especially if they are to be eaten raw, and all food should be stored according to instructions.

- **Salmonellosis:** *Salmonella* bacteria are particularly associated with poultry and eggs and therefore pregnant women should be particularly careful when handling these foods. Eggs should be cooked until both the white and the yolk are solid. Pasteurized egg products (either in the dry or liquid form) can be used in recipes requiring partially cooked or uncooked eggs. All meat, but particularly poultry, should be cooked thoroughly and raw meat should not be allowed to come into contact with or drip onto any other food.

- **Toxoplasmosis:** This is caused by a parasite found in raw meat, cat faeces and occasionally in goats' milk. In rare cases the infection can be passed on to an unborn baby and cause eye and brain damage. To avoid toxoplasmosis, pregnant women should not eat raw or uncooked meat, unpasteurized goats' milk or goats' cheese, or unwashed fruit and vegetables. After handling raw meat, chopping board, utensils and hands should be washed thoroughly. To protect against garden soil fouled by cats, rubber gloves should be worn when gardening and also when changing cat litter trays.

Practical solutions to nutritional problems

Low iron intake: Advise several portions of iron-rich foods daily (see page 7 and Part 1, pages 28–29), eaten together with a rich source of vitamin C to help absorption, for example orange juice, citrus fruit, green vegetables, peppers, tomatoes. Advise avoidance of bran and avoidance of tea at meal times.

Low calcium intake: Advise a minimum of half a pint of semi-skimmed milk daily or calcium-rich alternatives such as yogurt or cheese. For those unable to comply, advise a calcium-fortified soya milk. See Table 1.3 for other sources of calcium.

Poor weight gain: Advise increased consumption of foods selected from the four main groups (see Appendix 1 and Part 1, page 31). If appetite is poor, these foods can be eaten as snacks between meals, for example a sandwich, cheese and crackers, fruit, glass of milk, bowl of breakfast cereal. Advise whole milk instead of low fat milk. Ask about exercise pattern.

Excessive weight gain: Ask about dietary pattern and advise on swapping nutrient-rich foods for foods currently eaten that provide calories (energy) but little else, such as fruit instead of sweets and biscuits. Do not attempt to restrict weight gain or energy intake severely.

Atopic families and concern about allergy: There is some evidence that infants may be sensitized to food proteins which cross the placenta. However, the benefits of women avoiding specific foods during pregnancy are not proven (see page 18).

Lactation

Energy

The calculated energy cost of lactation is around 650 kcal per day but allowance must be made for the energy derived from weight loss. Thus, the additional average requirement for energy intake for mothers who breast feed exclusively for the first 3–4 months, followed by the progressive introduction of weaning foods, is about 500 kcal per day, corresponding to an average milk output of about 750 ml per day (DH, 1991).

Vitamins and minerals

Extra quantities of many essential nutrients are required to compensate for the amounts secreted into the milk each day. The requirement for extra nutrients should be met provided that energy intake is adequate and increased according to appetite, and provided that a varied selection of foods is chosen, especially those of high nutrient density. For information on specific nutrients, see Table 1.2 and pages 4–7 and 7–15.

Fluid

As the daily milk volume when the baby is 2–3 months may be as high as 820 ml, an adequate intake of fluid is obviously crucial for the maintenance of the supply of breast milk. A high fluid intake is also essential immediately post partum, when the mother is establishing breast feeding. The best guide to requirement is thirst and the forced drinking of extra liquid will not improve the quality or quantity of the milk.

Slimming

It is not advisable to reduce total food intake with a view to slimming during lactation, as this could result in a low intake of important nutrients. The mobilization of fat stores, although only gradual, may help mothers to reduce their weight. Women who are overweight at this stage should be given appropriate advice to enable them to base their diets on nutrient-dense foods (those with a high vitamin and mineral content in relation to calorie content) and to avoid excessive amounts of energy-dense, high fat, sugar-rich foods.

Influence of maternal diet on breast milk composition

Maternal diet has virtually no effect on the protein, total fat and energy composition of breast milk, though the fatty acid composition of the mother's diet will influence the fatty acid composition of the milk she produces. The latter may be important but the significance is yet to be established.

However, individual foods eaten by a mother may influence the composition of breast milk and in some cases lead to adverse reactions in her baby; for example, some mothers find that after eating spicy foods or onions, their babies experience abdominal discomfort. Obviously if this occurs, then those foods are best avoided, provided this does not result in omission of a number of foods considered to be important nutrient sources. In the same way alcohol should largely be avoided during breast feeding, because of the risk to the infant. Other non-nutritive substances which can pass into breast milk include caffeine, nicotine, senna and other amines and alkaloids. Excessive consumption of coffee, tea and cola drinks is reported to cause restlessness in some infants.

There is also evidence of sensitization to food proteins which cross the placenta or into breast milk. However, the benefits of the mother avoiding specific foods during pregnancy and lactation are not proven. Indeed it has been suggested that such exposure is important in establishing a normal immune response to these proteins. Because of the risk that the avoidance of groups of foods such as dairy products may lead to dietary imbalance, this procedure would only be recommended where the infant is seen to be markedly at risk as a result of a family history of atopy (Cant, 1991). See also Part 3, Food Intolerance and Allergy.

Drugs and breast feeding

Administration of some drugs to nursing mothers may be toxic to the baby if they are able to enter the milk in pharmacological quantities. Theoretically, even when concentrations are too low for a pharmacological effect, drugs are capable of causing hypersensitivity in an infant (for example, ergotamine), whereas others have little effect. Other drugs (for example, bromocriptine) inhibit lactation, or inhibit the infant's suckling reflex (for example, phenobarbitone).

For many drugs, there is currently insufficient information on potential effects during pregnancy and lactation to enable specific advice to be given, and consequently as a rule of thumb, drugs are best avoided during these periods. Where the use of drugs is essential, lists of drugs to be avoided or used with caution during pregnancy, and drugs which are excreted in breast milk, can be found in Appendix 4 and Appendix 5 of *MIMS*.

Recommended changes in policy

Research is indicating that diet before pregnancy, during pregnancy and breast feeding, and during infancy can have life-long effects on the health of the offspring. It is therefore of major importance that women are advised accordingly and that opportunities are taken to identify poorly nourished women before pregnancy and to give them specialist attention.

The following changes in practice and policy are recommended:

- Nutrition advice should be available for all women considering pregnancy, and the importance of preparing for pregnancy should be stressed. Advantage can be taken of existing clinics and services used by women of childbearing age.

- Particular attention should be paid to calcium and iron intakes prior to pregnancy, together with opportunistic measurement of iron stores. Advice on dietary iron should emphasize means of ensuring that iron is well absorbed as well as indicating dietary sources.

- Attention should be paid to appropriate weight gain during pregnancy. Particular concern should be attached to poor weight gain since new evidence indicates that good nutrition during pregnancy can help minimize the baby's chance of developing heart disease in middle age.

References

Barker DJP (Ed) (1992) *Fetal and Infant Origins of Adult Disease.* London, British Medical Journal.

Barker DJP et al. (1993) Growth in utero and serum cholesterol concentrations in adult life. *British Medical Journal* **307,** 1524–7.

Beattie JO (1992) Alcohol exposure and the fetus. *European Journal of Clinical Nutrition* **46,** (Suppl 1), S7–S17.

British Nutrition Foundation (1992) *Unsaturated Fatty Acids.* London, Chapman and Hall.

Bothwell TH et al. (1979) *Iron Metabolism in Man.* Oxford, Blackwell Scientific Publications. p. 576.

Briggs MH (1973) Cigarette smoking and infertility in men. *Medical Journal of Australia* **1,** 616–7.

Campbell DM (1983) Dietary restriction in obesity and its effect on neonatal outcome. In Campbell DM and Gillmer MDG (Eds) *Nutrition in Pregnancy.* Proceedings of the Tenth Study Group of the Royal College of Obstetricians and Gynaecologists. London, RCOG. pp 243–250.

Campbell DM (1991) Maternal and fetal nutrition. In McLaren DS et al. (Eds) *Textbook of Paediatric Nutrition.* 3rd edn. London, Churchill Livingstone. pp 3–20.

Cant AJ (1991) Food allergy and intolerance. In McLaren DS et al. (Eds) *Textbook of Paediatric Nutrition.* 3rd edn. London, Churchill Livingstone. pp 201–221.

Chief Medical Officer (1990) Women cautioned: watch your vitamin A intake. Press release no. 90/507. London, Department of Health.

Cockburn F et al. (1980) Maternal vitamin D intake and mineral metabolism in mothers and their new born infants. *British Medical Journal* **281,** 11–14.

Crawford MA et al. (1986) A comparison of food intake during pregnancy and birthweight in high and low socio-economic groups. *Progress in Lipid Research* **25,** 249–54.

Dawes MG et al. (1992) Routine weighing in pregnancy. *British Medical Journal* **304,** 487–9.

Department of Health, Committee on Medical Aspects of Food Policy (1991) *Dietary Reference Values for Food Energy and Nutrients in the United Kingdom. Report on Health and Social Subjects 41.* London, HMSO.

Department of Health (1992a) *Folic Acid and the Prevention of Neural Tube Defects.* Report from an Expert Advisory Group. Manchester, Health Publications Unit.

Department of Health (1992b) *While You Are Pregnant: Safe Eating and How to Avoid Infection from Food and Animals.* London, DH.

Dimperio DL et al. (1992) Routine weighing during antenatal visits: still justified. *British Medical Journal* **304,** 460.

Doyle W et al. (1982) Dietary survey during pregnancy in a low socio-economic group. *Human Nutrition: Clinical Nutrition* **39a,** 95–106.

Doyle W et al. (1989) Maternal nutrient intake and birthweight. *Journal of Human Nutrition and Dietetics* **2,** 415–22.

Evans HJ et al. (1981) Sperm abnormalities and cigarette smoking. *Lancet* **1,** 627–9.

Golding J et al. (1990) Factors associated with childhood cancer in a national cohort study. *British Journal of Cancer* **62,** 304–8.

Hambidge KM (1989) Mild zinc deficiency in human subjects. In Mills CF (Ed) *Zinc in Human Biology.* London, Springer-Verlag. pp 281–296.

Haste FM et al. (1991) The effect of nutritional intake on outcome of pregnancy in smokers and non-smokers. *British Journal of Nutrition* **65,** 347–54.

Hendry WF (1979) Male subfertility. *British Journal of Family Planning* **5,** 29–31; 58–61.

Himmelberger DU et al. (1978) Cigarette smoking during pregnancy and the occurrence of spontaneous abortion and congenital abnormality. *American Journal of Epidemiology* **108,** 470–9.

Jones KL et al. (1973) Pattern of malformation in offspring of chronic alcoholic mothers. *Lancet* **1,** 1267–71.

Lind T (1983) Iron supplementation during pregnancy. In Campbell DM and Gillmer MDG (Eds). *Nutrition in Pregnancy.* Proceedings of the Tenth Study Group of the Royal College of Obstetricians and Gynaecologists. London, RCOG. pp 181–191.

Lucas A et al. (1992) Breast milk and subsequent intelligence quotient in children born preterm. *Lancet* **339,** 261–4.

MRC Vitamin Study Research Group (1991) Prevention of neural tube defects: results of Medical Research Council Vitamin Study. *Lancet* **388,** 131–7.

Murray-Lyon I (1989) Alcohol and pregnancy. *Maternal and Child Health,* June, 165–9.

Office of Population Censuses and Surveys (1992) *1990 Mortality Statistics. Perinatal and Infant: Social and Biological Factors. England and Wales. Series DH3, No. 24.* London, HMSO.

Office of Population Censuses and Surveys (1993) *Health Survey for England*. London, HMSO.

Paulson SK and Deluca HF (1986) Vitamin D metabolism during pregnancy. *Bone* **7,** 331–6.

Rantakallio P (1978) The effect of maternal smoking on birthweight and subsequent health of the child. *Early Human Development* **2,** 371–82.

Royal College of Physicians (1987) *A Great and Growing Evil: The Medical Consequences of Alcohol Abuse*. London, Tavistock.

Schofield C et al. (1989) The diets of pregnant and postpregnant women in different social groups in London and Edinburgh: calcium, iron, retinol, ascorbic acid and folic acid. *British Journal of Nutrition* **62,** 363–77.

US National Academy of Medicine, Institute of Medicine (1990) *Nutrition During Pregnancy*. Washington, National Academy Press.

Wharton B (1992) Food and biological clocks. *Proceedings of the Nutrition Society* **51,** 145–53.

Wright JT et al. (1983) Alcohol and coffee consumption during pregnancy. In Campbell DM and Gillmer MDG (Eds) *Nutrition in Pregnancy*. Proceedings of the Tenth Study Group of the Royal College of Obstetricians and Gynaecologists. London, RCOG. pp 195–205.

Wynn M and Wynn A (1981) *The Prevention of Handicap of Early Pregnancy Origin. Some Evidence for the Value of Good Health Before Conception*. London, Foundation for Education and Research in Childbearing.

Wynn SW et al. (1994) The association of maternal social class with maternal diet and the dimensions of babies in a population of London women. *Nutrition and Health* **9,** 303–15.

Further reading

Buttriss J and Gray J (1994) *Maternal and Fetal Nutrition. Fact File 12*. London, National Dairy Council.

Buttriss J and Gray J (1995) *The Nutrition of Infants and Preschool Children. Fact File 2 (revised)*. London, National Diary Council.

Buttriss J and Hyman K (Eds) (1995) *The Growing Cycle: Child, Mother, Child*. Proceedings of a conference, 1994. London, National Diary Council.

Infant feeding and weaning

Key points

1. The evidence that breast milk is the best food for young infants is now overwhelming. Mothers should receive the necessary advice, support and encouragement to breast feed. The majority of women should be encouraged to breast feed up to at least four months and, ideally, beyond six months.

2. Although the incidence of breast feeding increased to 65% in 1980 from low levels in the 1960s, there has been no further increase over the past decade. In contrast, the incidence of breast feeding in some other Northern European countries is considerably greater.

3. To help achieve a better rate of breast feeding among mothers and improve infant feeding in general, a practice infant feeding policy could be devised. As well as strategies for increasing breast feeding, this could include an audit of the percentage of new-borns currently being breast fed, the age at which breast feeding is stopped or supplementary feeds introduced, and the age at which solids are introduced. Again, to help achieve a better rate of breast feeding, it is important that the feeding policy used in primary health care is consistent with that used in hospitals in the area.

4. A variety of infant formula milks, mainly based on modified cows' milk, are available for use by mothers who are unable or unwilling to breast feed. Appropriate advice and support should also be available for these mothers.

5. The majority of babies should not be given solid foods before four months, but most should be offered a mixed diet by six months of age. However, surveys show that the introduction of solid foods before three months is common, though it may be detrimental to the child's health.

6. Milk (breast or formula) continues to be an important source of nutrition during the weaning process. The Department of Health recommends the advantages of continuing breast or bottle feeding throughout the first year of life.

7. Cows' milk should not be given as the main type of milk (that is, the main drink) until one year of age because it is low in iron and some vitamins. When introduced, it should be in the form of whole, pasteurized milk. But from four months, for the majority of infants, small amounts of milk can be used to mix cereals and make custards and puddings. Other dairy products, such as yogurt and cheese, can also be introduced at this age.

8. Concern has been expressed about the iron intake of infants and young children. It is important that parents know which foods are good sources and of the need to establish these in their child's diet during the first year of life. In practice this means introducing iron-rich foods, such as meat, as well as iron-fortified foods, such as some breakfast cereals.

9. Vitamin supplements (A, C and D) are recommended from six months until at least two years of age for babies not given infant formula.

Infant feeding

Although the nutritional issues connected with infant feeding can appear complex, the basic principle is to ensure that the baby receives enough food of good quality. In practice, for infants under six months, this means supplying an adequate quantity of suitable milk, namely 120 ml/kg body weight.

For infants aged 6–12 months an adequate energy intake remains important to ensure that growth is maintained. About half of this should come from a suitable milk, and a minimum of 500 ml of breast milk or formula milk will be adequate. The other half of the child's energy intake should come from a variety of other foods, their consistency depending on the age of the child (see page 31).

It is crucial that advice given by health professionals is consistent. It is important, therefore, that all districts have an infant feeding policy, developed on a multi-disciplinary basis. This policy could usefully include strategies to promote breast feeding (see page 23).

The success or otherwise of infant nutrition is usually assessed against growth standards. There continues to be debate about the adequacy of current standards (Cole, 1993, 1994) but in general, longitudinal growth throughout infancy and early childhood should be monitored using appropriate charts. New charts have recently been developed (Freeman et al., 1995), which replace the old Tanner/Whitehouse standards developed in the 1950s and 1960s. The new charts are based on nine rather than seven centiles. Accompanying the new charts are recommendations for their use as referral tools. However, it should be recognized that breast-fed infants tend to be longer and thinner than those who are bottle fed.

It is essential in the early postnatal period that there is adequate monitoring of infant growth and support of the mother in feeding her baby. This should be undertaken initially by the midwives and subsequently by the health visitors, normally from day 11. However, the general practitioner has an opportunity to make further assessments at the time of the six-week postnatal examination and to discuss with the mother the importance of an appropriate feeding strategy to the long-term health of her child.

Trends in infant feeding

Detailed information on infant feeding practices in Great Britain has been collected in a series of surveys carried out by the Office of Population Censuses and Surveys in 1975, 1980, 1985 and 1990 (Martin, 1978; Martin and Monk, 1982; Martin and White, 1988; White et al., 1992).

The incidence of breast feeding reached an all time low in the 1960s by which time most women were giving birth in hospital. However, since then it has increased considerably from 51% of women in England and Wales in 1975 to 67% in 1980 (65% in the whole of Great Britain). Since the early 1980s, there has been little change.

In 1990, 63% of mothers in Great Britain started to breast feed (White et al., 1992). By six weeks, 39% of those who had started to breast feed had stopped. However, many more mothers are now giving supplementary bottles of infant formula to breast-fed babies so that by four weeks after birth, the majority of babies in Great Britain are receiving at least some infant formula feeds, and by four months three quarters appear to be fully bottle fed. The proportion of breast-fed babies who receive additional bottles at six weeks has risen from 28% in 1980 to 34% in 1985 and 39% in 1990.

In contrast, in Norway nearly all women breast feed their infants to start with, and 80% are still breast feeding at three months. Even at six months, 50% of infants are receiving breast milk and at a year this has fallen to 20% (National Nutrition Council, 1993).

In the 1990 OPCS survey, as in previous surveys, there was a strong influence of social class on the incidence of breast feeding: 89% of mothers of first babies in social class 1 compared with 50% of first time mothers in social class 5 (White et al., 1992). Women who are older at the birth of their first baby and those who have stayed in full-time education beyond 18 years of age are also more likely to breast feed. The duration of breast feeding is also influenced by various factors, so those who breast feed the longest tend to be from higher social classes and/or have been educated beyond the age of 18.

The Panel on Child Nutrition, Committee on Medical Aspects of Food Policy, reviewed current infant feeding practices and made recommendations (DHSS, 1988). This has been followed in 1994 by a new COMA report which concentrates specifically on weaning and diet for children under two years (DH, 1994).

Infant nutrient and fluid requirements

Dietary references values (DRVs) for energy and nutrients (DH, 1991) are given in Part 1 (Appendix 2). Unlike previous guidelines on nutrient intake, the new figures have been set for each of the four three-month periods of infancy.

The dietary reference values for younger infants are based on estimates from data for bottle-fed infants and are intended to be used only for assessing the diets of bottle-fed infants, as reference values for breast-fed infants would have no value in practice (DH, 1991). In some cases, the dietary reference values for infants aged 0–3 months who are fed infant formula are in excess of those which might be expected to be obtained from breast milk. This is because the efficiency of absorption of energy and some nutrients from formula milks is known to be less than that from breast milk.

Skeletal growth and development is rapid during the first year of life and this is reflected in the high calcium and phosphorus needs of infants compared with older children.

The intake of fluid will vary from day to day and between different infants. However, in general, babies drink about 150 ml of fluid per kilogram of body weight per day in the early months of life, decreasing to about 100 ml per kilogram per day in later infancy.

Breast feeding

Need for a revised strategy?

Health professionals have become too complacent about the decision of many mothers not to breast feed and need to consider a change in policy. There is no doubt that the best nutrition for healthy infants at term, and for the first few months, is breast milk. It is essential, therefore, that mothers should receive every possible encouragement to breast feed their babies (DHSS 1988; DH, 1991; Royal College of Midwives, 1991). Mothers should be encouraged to breast feed up to at least four months, and ideally beyond six months (DH, 1994).

Improving the incidence of breast feeding

There is a need for a change in policy, and specific multidisciplinary infant feeding policies which embrace the role of the hospital and the primary health care team need to be established. A starting point for developing such a policy (or establishing whether a policy already exists) is the local maternity services advisory committee.

The job of helping mothers to establish successful breast feeding falls increasingly to members of the practice team now that mothers often leave hospital 48 hours after the baby is born. This new situation may require a change in strategy and in the mode of management of the care of pregnant women and nursing mothers. At the same time, skills need to be acquired to ensure that women who are unable (in reality few are, given appropriate support) or unwilling to breast feed their baby are not made to feel guilty. Particular attention may need to be paid to encouraging mothers in lower socio-economic groups to breast feed (see page 22).

To help achieve a better rate of breast feeding

among mothers and to improve infant feeding in general, a practice strategy could be devised which dovetails with the infant feeding policy. As well as strategies for increasing breast feeding, this could include an audit of the percentage of new-borns currently being breast fed, the age at which breast feeding is stopped or supplementary feeds introduced, and the age at which solids are introduced, together with appropriate targets.

At the end of 1992, a new National Breast Feeding Working Group was established as part of the government's Health of the Nation initiative. This group is working in partnership with the UNICEF/WHO 'Baby Friendly Initiative' to ensure that the promotion of breast feeding in the UK is backed by both national and international efforts.

Helping to change women's views

Schools and antenatal clinics: Not only do many women never begin to breast feed, others give up very early. Strategies are needed to help overcome this. In order to encourage women to breast feed, appropriate information should be available early on, for example when girls are still at school. Adequate advice, support and encouragement should also be available through antenatal clinics throughout pregnancy, as detailed in a report of the Royal College of Midwives (1991). This could take the form of a discussion group featuring a mother from an appropriate ethnic and social group who actually demonstrates breast feeding. Men (and boys through school) should also be educated that breast feeding is best for the baby.

Local organizations: Local branches of organizations such as the National Childbirth Trust and the Baby Milk Action Coalition provide literature which can help to inform mothers-to-be of the advantages of breast milk for babies.

Active demonstrations of breast feeding: In many families there may be no recent practical knowledge of breast feeding. It may be helpful for women who are experienced in breast feeding actively to demonstrate the technique to other women, so as to remove some of the mystery.

Targeting groups where breast feeding incidence is commonly low: It may be important to address the needs for information and practical advice of certain subgroups in the practice population, for example low income families, particular ethnic groups. It is important that the target groups for such advice should be able to relate socially and ethnically to those giving advice.

Advice and support for breast-feeding mothers

The key points in establishing breast feeding are:

- demand feeding
- no supplementary feeding
- no supplementary drinks.

However, when giving general support to mothers who wish to breast feed, giving advice on the following factors have been shown to help:

Support at the first feed: The psychological impact of a mother's first breast-feeding experience is very important in terms of her feelings towards her baby and is also crucial to the continuance of breast feeding. In most cases the baby will be ready to feed within an hour of birth and it is the midwife's responsibility to ensure that mother and baby experience a satisfactory first feed. It is very important that advice and support is given at this crucial time and over the following days. *Successful Breastfeeding* (RCM, 1991) describes the sort of advice to be given, for example the composition of colostrum and mature milk, changing milk composition during a feed, the importance of correct positioning, an outline of the physiology of lactation and the baby's mechanism of milk removal, and the baby's likely feeding needs.

Unrestricted duration of feeds: There is no need to allow the baby to suckle for only a specified period of time.

Unrestricted frequency of feeds: The baby can be fed on demand, rather than at set times.

Feeding the baby at night: Milk production continues as efficiently at night as by day and if milk is not removed, the breasts will become engorged. This will cause discomfort but will also begin to suppress lactation. Feeding the baby at night will help to prevent this.

Reduced emphasis on the baby's weight gain: If too much emphasis is placed on this, mothers may feel that they are not able to satisfy their baby's need (particularly as it is not possible to see how much the baby has taken) and so decide to change to formula feeds where they can actually measure the volume consumed.

Breast feeding after caesarean section: Delivery by caesarean section does not preclude breast feeding. The mother should be warned that breast feeding will be painful because it causes abdominal contractions, and that particular care will be needed in the first few days with positioning the mother and baby — mothers are generally more comfortable feeding when they are lying down. The National Childbirth Trust produces a leaflet on the subject.

After the birth of twins: Most women can breast feed two babies successfully, though it does require additional time and determination. Correct positioning of the babies enables mothers to feed both babies simultaneously. Mothers of twins who are breast feeding are likely to become very tired and will need additional support with household tasks. The National Childbirth Trust produces a leaflet on the subject.

Advantages of breast feeding

More attention should be given to emphasizing the many advantages that breast feeding confers to both mother and infant. These include:

- Above all the **composition** of the milk is appropriate for the needs of the infant and the nutrients it contains are readily absorbed

- It confers considerable **protection against infection** not only because it is a clean source of food but because it contains various anti-infective agents including immunoglobulins, especially immunoglobulin A, lactoferrin, lysozyme, lymphocytes and macrophages

- It contains enzymes, hormones and other factors which may be important for **growth and development** of various organs, notably the gastro-intestinal tract.

- It is both **convenient** and **cheap**

- It enables the infant to **regulate its own food supply**

- It can promote **bonding** between mother and infant

- It aids **involution of the uterus** and may help in the **loss of surplus weight** by the mother.

- There is also evidence that exclusive breast feeding may help to **protect against:**

  — intolerance and allergies in infants with a family history of atopy
  — insulin dependent diabetes
  — impaired brain development, especially in premature infants who have been born too early to have stored the n-3 fatty acids necessary for development of brain structure (see page 29).

Breast feeding for the first six weeks may also confer long-lasting advantages to the health of the child, especially in relation to response to infection in childhood (Howie et al., 1990).

Nevertheless, women will have expectations that bottle feeding is more convenient, and arguments to counter these views need to be prepared; for example, women perceive that:

- Bottle-fed babies go for four hours between feeds but in the early stages, breast-fed infants may need feeds two-hourly. Parents need to understand that breast feeding is a full-time occupation and that it is likely to upset their normal lifestyle totally.

- Fathers can only play their part in caring for the baby if bottle feeding is chosen. This is not correct. There are a number of positive ways in which fathers can contribute towards caring for a breast-fed baby (apart from nappy changing), including comforting the baby and bringing the child to the mother whilst she is preparing to feed, and holding the baby and settling him or her down after feeding.

- It is not possible to breast feed twins simultaneously. In fact it is not only possible, but saves a good deal of time to feed twins simultaneously.

In addition, early discharge can be turned into an advantage — new mothers are more settled at home.

It is vital, therefore, that adequate support is given to the mother immediately after the birth and in the first week postnatally so that breast feeding, once initiated, can be maintained. This support should be provided by midwives in hospitals and in the community, and later by health visitors and general practitioners (RCM, 1991). Above all, there is a need for consistency of advice.

Why women stop breast feeding

It is also important to consider why women stop breast feeding. These factors can form a useful basis for a strategy designed to encourage breast feeding. Reasons include the following:

- In the OPCS surveys, 'insufficient milk' was the most common reason reported by mothers for stopping breast feeding earlier than planned. In fact, true failure of lactation is rare. If a breast-fed baby appears hungry, the first response should be to breast feed more often. The mother may need a lot of encouragement and support, and to be reassured that if she feeds her baby according to demand, her milk supply will increase to meet the baby's needs.

- Supplementary and complementary bottle feeding, or 'topping-up' with infant formula feeds, has not been shown to be of any benefit to healthy, full-term babies and is a major cause of hindering the establishment and maintenance of breast feeding. Furthermore, the baby can become confused by the difference in technique between suckling on a bottle and suckling at the breast and hence feed less well. Replacement of a breast feed by a bottle feed is likely to reduce milk production because of reduced breast stimulation. The mother may then begin to doubt whether she can produce enough milk for her baby and turn to bottle feeding for the reassurance of seeing how much her baby consumes.

- If a baby does not seem to be satisfied by breast feeds, another possible explanation is that the baby is not well positioned at the breast and so cannot obtain the milk. Particularly in the early days of establishing breast feeding, mothers may need help to make sure that the baby is properly latched onto the breast, and that the mother herself is comfortable enough to feed for as long as her baby needs. For detailed information abut the physiology and technique of breast feeding, refer to *Successful Breastfeeding* (RCM, 1991).

- The mother's lifestyle (for example, the need to return to work early) may make breast feeding difficult. Expressing breast milk may be a solution, and breast pumps can be hired, for example from local branches of the National Childbirth Trust.

What are the alternatives?

Mothers should be helped to make informed decisions about infant feeding by the provision of appropriate information before and during pregnancy, but it is important that they should not be made to feel guilty if they choose to bottle feed. It must be recognized that for some women the decision may not be easy or straightforward. Whatever a woman's decision, it should be respected and supported. Bottle feeding (see pages 27–30) can provide a nutritionally acceptable alternative for mothers who are unable or unwilling to breast feed, and parents choosing this method also need adequate advice and support about appropriate formulae and feed preparation.

Dealing with mastitis

There is no justification for advising a mother with mastitis to stop breast feeding. Indeed, abrupt weaning appears to increase the chances of a breast abscess (RCM, 1991).

Non-infective mastitis is often a consequence of engorgement and should be prevented in the same way, by demand feeding day and night. It also helps to ensure that the baby is correctly attached on each feeding occasion and the 'let-down' reflex effectively stimulated. Localized obstructions in the breast tissue should be avoided by the woman not wearing clothing that puts pressure on the breasts, gentle handling of the breasts to avoid bruising, not gripping the breast tightly when supporting it during feeding, and treating lumpiness by encouraging drainage from that area (improving position and stroking the affected area towards the nipple).

Infective mastitis can be caused by bacterial infection following damage to the epithelium of the breast or nipple. This can result from incorrect positioning of the baby at the breast or a reaction to a cream, lotion or spray.

Provided it is possible to monitor the mother closely, it may be possible to delay antibiotic treatment for 6–8 hours, whilst taking the corrective measures described above. However, if this is not possible, a broad spectrum antibiotic is the normal treatment. Most types do not appear in the breast milk in sufficient amounts to affect the baby.

Giving additional fluids

Supplementary feeds of infant formula to breast-fed infants can hinder the establishment and maintenance of breast feeding (see above). Provision of water or glucose/dextrose solutions is also unnecessary, even in hot weather (see page 33).

Infant formula milks

Milks designated as infant formulae should be suitable for babies from birth onwards and their composition is governed by a number of directives and guidelines (Table 2.1). Most infant formulae used in the UK are sold as a dried powder, but many companies now also market ready-to-feed milks available either in a glass bottle or a laminated carton. The Department of Health recommends that powdered milk feeds are reconstituted in a standard way by adding one scoopful of powder to each 30 ml (1 fluid ounce) of water. It is important that parents are aware that they should not pack down the powder into the scoop, causing an over-concentrated feed. This standard dilution is suitable from birth.

Standard milks

Two types of standard infant milk are available. Whey-dominant milks are based on dialysed whey protein (from cows' milk). Casein-dominant milks are based on whole cows' milk protein. Table 2.2 shows the

Table 2.1 *Compositional guidelines for infant milks (per 100ml)*

	DHSS (1980)	†ESPGAN (1977)	EEC (1991)★
Protein (g)	1.2–2.0	1.2–1.9	
whey			1.2–2.0
casein			1.5–2.0
Fat (g)	2.3–5.0	2.7–4.1	2.2–4.4
Carbohydrate (g)	4.8–10.0	5.4–8.2	4.7–9.4
Energy (kcal)	65–75	64–72	60–75
(kj)	270–310	270–300	250–310
Sodium (mmol)	0.6–1.5	0.6–1.2	0.5–1.9
Calcium (mg)	30–120	min 40	min 32
Iron (mg)	0.07–0.7	min 0.7	0.32–1.2

Source: Adapted from Lawson (1992).

★*Statutory Instrument No. 77, The Infant Formula and Follow-on Formula Regulations 1995*, was laid before Parliament in January 1995 and came into force in March 1995. These Regulations implement the EEC Directive 91/321/EEC referred to here.

†ESPGAN = European Society for Paediatric Gastroenterology and Nutrition.

Table 2.2 *Composition of standard formulae (per 100ml)*

	Whey dominant				Casein dominant					
	Nutricia Premium	SMA Gold	Farley First	Milupa Aptamil	Nutricia Plus	SMA White	Farley Second	Milupa Milumil	Cows' milk	Breast milk
Protein (g)	1.4	1.5	1.5	1.5	1.9	1.5	1.7	1.9	3.3	1.3
Fat (g)	3.6	3.6	3.8	3.6	3.4	3.6	2.6	3.1	4.0	4.1
Carbohydrate (g)	7.5	7.2	7.0	7.3	7.3	7.2	8.6	8.4	4.7	7.2
Energy (kcal)	66	65	68	67	66	65	65	69	67	69
(kj)	275	270	285	280	275	270	270	290	280	290
Sodium (mg)	0.8	0.6	0.8	0.8	1.1	0.8	1.1	1.0	57	15
Calcium (mg)	54	42	35	59	86	46	61	71	119	34
Iron (mg)	0.5	0.6	0.6	0.7	0.5	0.6	0.6	0.4	0.05	0.07

Source: Adapted from Lawson (1992).

composition of brands available in the UK. For comparison, the composition of cows' milk and breast milk are also given.

A number of modifications are made to cows' milk. The concentrations of protein and minerals are reduced, lactose is increased by the addition of lactose or maltodextrins, and vitamins and trace elements are added so as to offer similar amounts as provided by breast milk.

In addition, the nature of the protein in the whey-dominant milk is changed from the casein:whey ratio of 80:20 found in cows' milk and casein-dominant formula to a ratio of 40:60, and vegetable oils are substituted for all or part of the milk fat.

Usually infants begin on a whey-dominant formula. However, there is no evidence that this is more beneficial than a casein-dominant milk, although the higher calcium: phosphorus ratio in whey-dominant milks may be more appropriate for very young babies.

There is a commonly held belief that casein-dominant milks are more satisfying for the older 'hungrier' baby but a recent study failed to substantiate this belief (Taitz and Scholey, 1989).

An adequate substitute for breast milk?

All formulae lack the immunological and anti-infective properties of breast milk and the many other factors listed earlier (page 25). Nevertheless, it is clear that infants on breast milk have a different growth trajectory from that of bottle-fed infants. However, the modern cows' milk formulae have been developed to mimic human milk as clearly as is technologically feasible at present, and in the light of current knowledge. So in terms of overall nutrient composition, the differences between formulae and breast milk are now relatively small. This is especially so in the most highly modified formulae, which are based on whey protein and in which the fat is predominantly provided as polyunsaturated and monounsaturated fatty acids.

As research provides more information on the significance of the various factors in breast milk, there is no doubt that manufacturers will continue to improve the composition of infant formulae. For example, the importance of the high levels of taurine in human milk is not as yet fully understood, although taurine has a role in brain and retinal development as well as in bile salt composition. However, some formulae do now contain added taurine.

Recent research has confirmed in practical

Table 2.3 *Recommendations and composition of pre-term formulae (per 100 ml)*

| | Recommendations †ESPGAN (1987) | Composition of pre-term formulae | |
	For use in hospital	Hospital, ready-to-feed	For home use
Protein (g)	1.8–2.5	2.0–2.2	1.8–2.0
Fat (g)	2.9–5.6	3.4–4.9	3.5–4.1
Carbohydrate (g)	5.6–11.2	7.0–8.6	7.2–7.7
Energy (kcal)	65–85	68–80	70–74
(kj)	270–335	285–335	293–310
Sodium (mmol)	0.6–1.5	0.9–1.83	0.96–1.17
Iron (mg)	1.9–2.5 mg/kg/day max 15 mg/day	0.04–0.9	0.07–0.65

Source: Adapted from Lawson (1992).
†ESPGAN = European Society for Paediatric Gastroenterology and Nutrition.

terms the importance of essential fatty acids of both the n-6 series (precursor linoleic acid) and the n-3 series (precursor alpha-linolenic acid) and their long chain metabolites in cell structure and organ growth and development (Farquharson et al., 1992; Lucas et al., 1992). In particular, they are needed for the structural development of the brain during gestation and early childhood, and it has been suggested that inadequate provision may affect subsequent IQ. These long chain fatty acids are found in breast milk and are now being added to some infant formulae; however the optimum amount needed by term infants remains unclear.

Pre-term infants

Babies born prematurely, like all low birth-weight babies, require extra nutrients for rapid growth. But pre-term infants are at a particular nutritional disadvantage because they have missed the period of maximum transfer of energy and nutrients from mother to fetus during the last months of pregnancy. In addition, the immature state of gastro-intestinal and renal function results in poor absorption and reduced retention of nutrients.

Premature infants are usually discharged from hospital at a weight at or below 2 kg. Up until this time they will usually have received either a pre-term formula, the recommended composition of which is shown in Table 2.3,

or a combination of breast milk and pre-term formula. Ordinary infant milks are not normally used.

Typically following discharge, pre-term infants will be fed on a standard infant formula or breast milk. A number of formulae designed for feeding the pre-term infant are now available in powder and ready-to-feed format for use in the community. The need for these formulae remains somewhat controversial, but they may be recommended for use until the infant is 2.5–3.0 kg in weight. They are available on request from retail chemists, but milk tokens cannot be used for these formulae.

Pre-term formulae have a higher nutrient density than standard milks, providing more energy, protein and sodium per 100 ml. The mineral, trace element and vitamin content has also been modified to take into account the higher nutrient requirements of such infants.

Even after discharge, pre-term infants will require iron and vitamin supplements. With an increasing number of very premature infants surviving, it may be necessary to establish, with local paediatricians a protocol for management of these babies once they have left hospital.

Weaning onto solids is normally acceptable once the baby weighs at least 5 kg, has lost the extrusion reflex and is able to eat from a spoon (DH, 1994).

Weaning

When to wean

Most health authorities now have a food and health policy for the under fives which includes key nutritional recommendations about weaning. A copy can usually be obtained from the community dietitian or hospital-based paediatric dietitian, although these may require updating in the light of the government's new report on weaning (DH, 1994).

Weaning becomes necessary to:

- meet the changing nutritional needs of the growing infant
- encourage the development of the ability to bite and chew
- encourage the transition to family foods.

The Department of Health advises that most babies do not need solid foods (anything other than breast or formula milks) before four months of age but the majority of babies should be offered a mixed diet not later than the age of six months (DH, 1994). The premature introduction of solids is undesirable for several reasons. Before the age of four months, babies find it difficult to pass food from the front to the back of their mouths and some infants do not readily develop the ability to bite and to chew solid foods or are not willing to experiment with foods of different flavours, textures and consistency. The gut is more vulnerable to infection and to allergy and the use of energy-dense foods may facilitate obesity. In breast-fed babies, the superior bioavailability of nutrients such as iron may be compromised by anything other than exclusive breast feeding in the early months.

Late weaning (after six months) is also inadvisable — babies sometimes find it more difficult to accept solids, as important developmental stages have been missed. Also nutritional status may be compromised.

During the last few weeks of gestation, babies build up a reserve of nutrients sufficient to support growth for the first few months of life. For example, iron stores become depleted after about six months of breast feeding. The introduction of suitable weaning foods may therefore determine whether these low iron stores progress to frank iron deficiency (Oski and Landow, 1980) and its complications which, apart from anaemia, may also include impairment of psychomotor function and defects in cellular immunity (Dallman, 1986). See page 44 and Part 1, (page 29) for dietary sources of iron.

Trends in weaning and mixed feeding

The early introduction of solids is still common in Britain, although it has fallen during the last 15 years. In the 1990 OPCS survey, 19% of mothers had introduced solids before 10 weeks of age, although by the time the baby was three months old 68% of mothers had introduced solids (White et al., 1992). Most babies do not need solids before four months.

Therefore many mothers appear to be starting to wean their infants before it is considered to be advisable. In all surveys, bottle-fed babies were more likely to receive solids at an early age than breast-fed babies and, as with bottle feeding, there was a gradient of earlier introduction of solids down the social class structure.

Data on the food and nutrient intake of infants aged 6–12 months have been collected by the Ministry of Agriculture, Fisheries and Food (MAFF) (Mills and Tyler, 1992). This survey provides further evidence of early weaning patterns; over 50% of infants had received some solid food by 12 weeks of age. The infants were consuming a wide range of foods and, as might be expected, variety increased with increasing age. Commercial weaning foods formed a large part of the diet of most infants and few relied on 'family foods' alone, especially in the younger infants (6–9 months).

One notable finding was that iron intake may

be marginal in the second half of infancy (6–12 months), especially in older infants and in those fed 'family foods', and where breast milk, cows' milk and low fat milks are the main types of milk drunk.

Suitable weaning foods

Milk (breast or infant formula) remains important during weaning; even at one year of age the child will still be receiving half its energy intake as milk. As a baby's intake of food increases, the amount of milk required will decrease. However, milk remains an important staple in a child's diet and an intake of at least a pint (but no more than 2 pints) should be maintained up to the age of one year to maintain energy and calcium intake. After this age, a minimum of 350 ml of milk (usually cows' milk) is needed to meet calcium requirements (for information on suitable milks, see page 34).

An adequate energy intake is important and mothers need to know about the importance of iron and vitamins D and C in particular for this age group, and the foods in which these nutrients are found (see Part 1, Appendix 2).

There are no hard and fast rules. Table 2.4, based on information provided in the 1994 COMA report on weaning (DH, 1994) gives useful guidelines for feeding infants from four months onwards. Before this, babies ideally receive breast milk. Alternatively, they should be given an infant formula. No other foods or drinks are usually necessary.

Most foods can be tried from four months, but:

- Babies should not be given chilli and spices (though mildly spiced foods will usually be tolerated).

- Sugar and salt should not be added to infants' foods — they are unnecessary.

- Whole nuts should not be given — they may cause choking.

- Because of concerns about salmonella, soft boiled eggs should be avoided; eggs should be cooked until both the yolk and white are solid (see Chapter 14).

- Pâté and soft cheese (such as Brie, Camembert) are not recommended for children under one year (cottage cheese, curd cheese, hard cheese such as Cheddar are fine) (see Chapter 14).

Once a baby is four months old, the following foods are good ones to try: vegetable or fruit purées (for example potato, carrot, yam, plantain, broccoli, apple, banana), non-wheat infant cereals, thin porridge (made from rice, cornmeal, sago, millet, tapioca), puréed lentils (dahl), and mild spices may be used. Once a baby is used to taking food from a spoon, the range of foods offered can be expanded to include custard or plain (unsweetened) yogurt, and well-puréed meat.

Commercial baby foods (tins, jars and packet foods) are by no means essential but can be convenient. They are also perfectly wholesome and nourishing, and dried foods can be particularly useful during the first few weeks when the quantity of food eaten is very small. But home-prepared early weaning foods such as puréed fruit and vegetables can be prepared in bulk and quickly frozen in clean ice cube trays to provide easily defrosted, small individual portions.

Commercial foods are also reassuring for mothers who lack cooking facilities or adequate cooking skills though they are more expensive. These factors are reflected in the large proportion of mothers who use commercially produced foods (see page 30).

Many commercial weaning foods are fortified with iron and in the MAFF survey the iron intake of those infants fed solely commercial foods was greater than that of those fed predominantly 'family foods' (Mills and Tyler, 1992). Some commercial baby foods, such as rusks, cereals and some ready-meals, are of particular importance for breast-fed infants because they are fortified with iron (see page 33).

There is clearly a need for more advice on suitable iron sources in the weaning diet. A

Table 2.4 *Recommendations for introducing a mixed diet*

4–6 months: A minimum of 600 ml breast milk or infant formula daily. The following foods can be introduced after 4 months: low fibre cereals (e.g. rice based), mashed/puréed starchy vegetables, smooth purée of soft cooked vegetables or fruit, cows' milk products (e.g. plain unsweetened yogurt, unsweetened custard, cheese sauce), soft cooked meat or pulses, low sugar desserts. The first foods offered should be of a smooth consistency and bland taste. This first stage may be short or may last several weeks, depending on the individual baby.

6–9 months: Once a variety of food is accepted from a spoon 2–3 times a day, reduce the amount of milk to 500–600 ml of breast milk, infant formula or follow-on formula daily. Cows' milk can now be used to mix solids and hard cheese is suggested as a 'finger food'. Starchy foods (2–3 servings daily): start to introduce some wholemeal bread and cereals, for example toast as a 'finger food'. Cooked vegetables and fruit can be coarser in texture or can be given raw as finger foods (2 servings daily from this group). Meat and meat alternatives (1 serving daily): soft cooked minced or puréed meat, fish or pulses. Chopped hard-boiled eggs can be given as a finger food. Encourage savoury foods rather than sweet ones. Provision of finger foods is important in helping develop self-feeding.

9–12 months: This stage is marked by a move to three meals a day, interspersed by snacks and/or drinks. The advice regarding milks and milk products remains the same. Daily servings of starchy foods should be increased to 3–4 and can be of normal adult texture. Wholemeal products should be encouraged and foods with added sugar (e.g. biscuits, cakes) should be discouraged. Servings of fruit/vegetables should be increased to 3–4 daily, and dilute unsweetened orange juice (for vitamin C) can be given with meals, especially if they are meat free. From the meat and alternatives group, a minimum of one food of 'animal' source or two of vegetable source should be given. Moderate amounts of butter or margarine can be given and small amounts of jam (if necessary) on bread. Try to limit salty foods. Finger foods remain important.

After 1 year: A minimum of 350 ml of milk or 2 servings of dairy products. Encourage a cup rather than a bottle. Whole cows' milk can be given as a main drink and soft cheeses, such as Brie, can be given (if used as a normal part of the family diet). Lower fat milks can be used in cooking, but not as a main drink. Starchy foods: at least one serving at each mealtime. Discourage high fat foods such as pastry. Fruit and vegetables: minimum of 4 servings daily, generally of an adult texture. To help iron absorption, give a good source of vitamin C at each meal. Meat and alternatives: encourage low fat meat and oily fish. Liver pâté can now be used. Limit crisps and savoury snacks — give bread or fruit if the child is hungry between meals. Do not add sugar to drinks and try to limit soft drinks (e.g. squash, fruit juice) to mealtimes. Encourage a pattern of three main meals a day, with 2–3 snacks in between (discourage frequent snacking on fatty or sugary foods).

Source: Buttriss JL and Gray J (1995). Adapted from Department of Health (1994).

list of suitable iron-rich weaning foods is given on page 34, and additional information can be found in Part 1, Appendix 2 and Part 3, Anaemia in Adults and Children.

At this early stage, the food should usually be in the form of a sloppy purée and should be offered before milk feeds on first one and then two occasions in the day. Once the child becomes accustomed to eating food from a spoon, a wider variety of foods can be introduced, including purées of lean meat, fish or poultry, whole cows' milk as a mixer for cereals and milk puddings, grated cheese, yogurt, fromage frais, cottage cheese, eggs, smooth nut and seed pastes such as smooth peanut butter or tahini. Sweetened foods and puddings should be avoided until bland and savoury foods are accepted.

The importance of dietary variety should not be underestimated, even during weaning. For example, the long chain n-3 fatty acids and their precursors are found only in a limited range of foods, such as oily fish and vegetables, but they are essential for the rapid brain development occurring during early childhood.

Gradually, the texture can move towards a mashed and then a chopped consistency. During the later stages of this process, crisp finger foods such as carrots and pieces of bread can be introduced as teeth erupt. Other suitable finger foods are suggested in Table 2.4.

By one year of age, a child should have progressed to eating three meals a day plus two to three suitable snacks in between (avoiding sugary or fatty snack foods).

Parents may need reassurance about the suitability of ordinary family food for their baby and information about how it can be prepared appropriately.

Quite naturally, a mother can become very concerned about feeding her baby and weaning can create particular anxiety. If a mother is concerned that her child is not eating enough, there is probably no real reason for concern if the baby is gaining weight, although the relationship between mother and child may need consideration. It is important that parents acknowledge that there is a large variation in growth rates from one baby to another.

If the child is failing to gain weight, however, investigation of the baby may be required. In infants under six months, further investigation is warranted if they fail to gain weight for one month or fail to gain at least 1 kg over a two-month period. Infants between six months and a year should be investigated if there is no weight gain for six weeks or they fail to gain at least 0.6 kg over a two-month period.

From the age of six months, a cup rather than a feeder beaker can be introduced for milk feeds, in preparation for a move away from bottle feeds by 12 months of age. Bottles should never be left propped in babies' mouths, as this can cause choking and dental decay (see page 148). This is particularly important from a dental health point of view if the child is receiving soya formula (see page 36) (DH, 1994).

Suitable sources of iron for weaning

Iron intake by some infants is of current concern, particularly as iron deficiency anaemia during infancy has been linked with growth impairment, compromised cellular immunity, and impaired intellectual development and performance (Fairweather-Tait, 1992; Walter, 1993). Iron needs can be met by use of suitable baby milks. However, this will not guarantee longer term iron adequacy of the preschool diet as it may conceal poor weaning practices.

It is essential that mothers are aware of suitable food sources of iron and accustom their infants to these foods before the 'safety net' of formula or follow-on milk is removed. Table 2.5 gives examples of family food and special baby foods which provide iron. For reference, the iron reference nutrient intake for infants aged 6–12 months is 7.8 mg per day. This falls to 6.9 mg per day for children aged 1–3 years.

It is important that non-meat sources of iron are given in combination with foods rich in vitamin C, such as citrus fruit and green vegetables, to help aid iron absorption. Tea and coffee, particularly at meals, hinder iron absorption (DH, 1994).

Water and drinks other than milk

A milk suitable for the child's age, and water, should constitute the main drinks. Other drinks should usually be confined to mealtimes and because of the risk to dental health, they should not be given in a feeding bottle or at bedtime (DH, 1994).

As long as the diet contains fruit and vegetables to provide vitamin C, there is no particular advantage in giving fruit juice instead of milk.

From six months of age, babies can be given boiled, unflavoured tap water; it is not needed before this age.

Bottled water also needs to be boiled and again is not needed by children under six months. Indeed, as it can have a high sodium

Table 2.5 *Examples of foods containing iron*

Family foods	Quantity	Iron (mg)
Iron well absorbed:		
Minced beef	50 g (3 tbsp)	1.4
Liver	50 g (3 tbsp)	5.0
Lamb	50 g (3 tbsp)	0.9
Pork	50 g (3 tbsp)	0.7
Chicken	50 g (3 tbsp)	0.4
Sausage	1 small	0.5
Meat paste	10 g	0.2
Corned beef	30 g	0.9
Sardines	50 g (2)	2.3
Fish fingers	60 g (2)	0.5
Iron less well absorbed:		
Lentils (cooked)	50 g (2 tbsp)	1.7
Baked beans (or other cooked beans)	50 g (1–2 tbsp)	0.7
Egg	40 g (1)	0.8
Green vegetables, e.g. beans, cabbage peas, courgette, sweetcorn	50 g (2–3 tbsp)	0.3–0.7
Dried fruit, e.g. apricot, raisins, dates	50 g (3 tbsp)	1–1.7
Avocado	50 g (3 tbsp)	0.2
Bread	1 slice	0.5–0.9
Digestive biscuit	1 large	0.4
Fortified/infant foods		
Rusk	18 g (1 large)	2.5–3.0
Weetabix	20 g (1)	1.5
Cornflakes	20 g	1.3
Rice Krispies	20 g	1.3
Iron-fortified jars of baby food	Stage 1: a jar	2.5
	Stage 2: a jar	3.5
Unfortified jars	Stage 1: a jar	1.0
	Stage 2: a jar	1.3
Dried baby foods	10 g (1 tbsp)	0.5
Infant formula	150 ml	1.0
Follow-on milk	150 ml	2.0

content, it is less suitable than ordinary tap water. Effervescent waters are not suitable (DH, 1994).

Milks considered suitable in the first year of life

Breast milk and infant formulae
The Department of Health (1994) stresses the advantage of continuing breast or bottle feeding throughout the first year. It also indicates that pasteurized cows' milk can be introduced from the age of four months — in cooked dishes such as custards and yogurt — and in small amounts to mix cereals after six months. But the low iron content of cows' milk means that it is best not to introduce this as a **main drink** (as opposed to being used in cooking and with cereal), until one year of age.

The MAFF survey showed that 29% of infants aged 6–12 months received infant formula, and whole cows' milk was consumed by almost two-thirds (Mills and Tyler, 1992). Breast milk was the sole source of milk for 7% of infants and a further 7% received breast milk in addition to other milks. Contrary to Department of Health advice, 5% of

Table 2.6 *Recommendations and compositions of follow-on formulae (per 100 ml)*

	Recommendations					
	†ESPGAN (1981)	EEC (1991)★	SMA Progress	Farley Junior	Boots Milk Drink	Cow & Gate Step Up
Protein	2.0–3.7	1.3–3.6	2.5	2.0	2.1	1.8
Fat (g)	2–4	2.0–5.2	2.8	3.0	3.4	3.8
Carbohydrate (g)	5.7–8.6	4.2–11.2	28.0	8.0	6.4	7.2
Energy (kcal)	65–85	60–80	65	67	65	70
(kj)	270–355	250–335	270	280	270	295
Sodium (mmol)	0.7–2.5	0.8–2.3	1.3	1.3	1.3	1.0
Iron (mg)	0.7–1.4	0.6–1.6	1.2	0.7	0.8	1.3
Vitamin D (µg)	0.7–1.4	0.6–2.4	1.2	1.1	1.3	2.1

Source: Adapted from Lawson (1992).   †ESPGAN = European Society for Paediatric Gastroenterology and Nutrition

★ *Statutory Instrument No. 77, The Infant Formula and Follow-on Formula Regulations 1995*, was laid before Parliament in January 1995, and came into force in March 1995. These Regulations implement the EEC Directive 91/321/EEC referred to here.

infants were receiving low fat milks as the main type of milk.

Follow-on formulae

These milks are based on cows' milk and are generally less modified than standard formulae. In the UK, they are considered suitable from six months of age. Compositional guidelines and the composition of some brands on the market are shown in Table 2.6. Follow-on milks cannot be exchanged for milk tokens.

The energy density of these milks is similar to standard formula but the protein content is higher. They are fortified with vitamins and trace elements, and the iron content is significantly higher than in standard formulae.

There is controversy about their use. They are marketed as a solution to iron deficiency anaemia and yet for most infants, a standard formula is adequate and there is no nutritional advantage in changing to this type of milk. However, they do provide the sense of progression for which some mothers feel a need. Where weaning has been delayed through developmental retardation or cultural preference, using a follow-on milk as a main drink may be of advantage because of its higher iron content.

In addition, concern has been expressed recently about the provision of large amounts of iron in diets of young children who have **adequate** iron stores (Idjradinata et al., 1994). There was evidence of reduced growth rate. The form of iron used to fortify infant foods is of relatively low bioavailability, and so large amounts need to be added to ensure needs are met. It used to be assumed that the extra iron which was not absorbed would pass harmlessly through the gut; however, this is now being questioned.

Milk and feeding problems

Automatically changing a baby's milk in response to a reported feeding problem is not the best course of action. However, there are times when appropriate investigation indicates that the method of feeding currently employed is not in the child's best interest. In such circumstances, various options are available, as discussed below.

Soya formulae

There are a number of formulae based on soya but modified for infants (Table 2.7). These are made from isolated soya protein (not whole soya beans) and are supplemented with methionine, carnitine, minerals, vitamins

Table 2.7 *Recommendations and compositions of soya formulae (per 100 ml)*

	Recommendations		Composition		
	†ESPGAN (1981)	EEC (1991)★	Nutricia Infasoy	SMA Wysoy	Farley Ostersoy
Protein (g)	1.3–2.2	1.7–2.0	1.8	1.8	1.9
Fat (g)	2.6–4.8	n/s	3.6	3.6	3.8
Carbohydrate (g)	5.2–9.6	n/s	7.1	6.9	7.0
Energy (kcal)	65–80	n/s	66	65	70
Calcium/phosphorus ratio	1.0–2.0:1	1.2–2.0:1	2.6:1	1.8:1	2.0:1
Iron/zinc ratio	2.5:1	n/s (0.7–1/1:1)	1.0:1	1.1:1	1.2:1

Source: Adapted from Lawson (1992).

†ESPGAN = European Society for Paediatric Gastroenterology and Nutrition

★ *Statutory Instrument No. 77, The Infant Formula and Follow-on Formula Regulations 1995* was laid before Parliament in January 1995 and came into force in March 1995. These Regulations implement the EEC Directive 91/321/EEC referred to here.

and trace elements, so that the available nutrients are similar to those in human milk. Formulae available in the UK are all free of lactose and are powders that are reconstituted in the same way as normal feeds — 1 scoopful per 30 ml (1 fluid ounce) of water.

Available through supermarkets and other shops, there are a number of soya drinks which are less modified and are **not** suitable for infants under the age of one. If consumed by preschool children, it is essential that they are accompanied by a good mixed diet and supplements of calcium and vitamins A, C and D.

Soya formulae can be prescribed by a general practitioner for proven milk intolerance and can also be purchased over the counter. Infant soya formulae are a vital part of the diet of children of vegan families who wish to avoid using animal products. However, their use in the prevention or treatment of suspected milk allergy is less clear. Many infants who are intolerant to cows' milk are also intolerant to soya protein (Eastham et al., 1982; Rennie, 1988; DH, 1994) and the allegation that soya formulae are less allergenic than cows' milk has not been confirmed, according to a joint report of the Royal College of Physicians and British Nutrition Foundation (1984). (See also Part 3, Food Intolerance and Allergy, and Malabsorption in Infants.)

The use of soya formulae from birth for infants of atopic families in order to prevent the onset of allergic symptoms has not been proved to be beneficial.

Where milk allergy is suspected and has been investigated, treatment should be managed by a paediatrician and a dietitian in order to ensure that the diet is nutritionally complete.

In order to avoid the use of lactose, other sugars, such as glucose and sucrose which are more cariogenic, are used. For this reason, it is particularly important that infants given such formulae progress quickly to a cup after six months (DH, 1994). Bottles and feeder cups both enable the teeth to be bathed in the potentially cariogenic milk. In particular, bottles should never be left propped in babies' mouths.

Goats' and sheep's milk
Goats' milk has been advocated for infants and children with suspected intolerance to cows' milk and, more recently, sheep's milk has become available. Both are unsuitable for infants under a year because of their high protein and sodium content, and deficiency of iron and vitamins A, C, D and folic acid.

Recently, a powdered goats' milk has become available which has been adapted for infants. When reconstituted, its composition meets current recommendations and is suitable for use after six months. However, a disadvantage is that the method of reconstitution (1 scoop per 50 ml) is different from that for other milks and so could cause confusion and the over-concentration of feeds.

Goats' milk is not currently included in EC legislation, so the availability of suitable products for infants after the implementation of the new regulations is unclear.

The similarity of the proteins found in different milks means that a high proportion of infants who react to cows' milk protein will also react to goats' or sheep's milk (DH, 1994).

Hydrolysed protein formulae
These formulae are usually based on cows' milk in which the protein has been broken down into simpler short chain peptides, which are much less allergenic. Such preparations are usually well tolerated by infants with a milk allergy and are available only on prescription for proven milk allergy. At present there is no evidence that early avoidance of cows' milk and feeding a hydrolysate will prevent allergy (Lawson, 1992).

Vitamin supplements

The Department of Health recommends that vitamin supplementation should be given to infants who are not formula fed from six months upwards. Supplements should be continued to at least two years and preferably five years. The daily dose should be:

Vitamin A	200 µg
Vitamin C	20 mg
Vitamin D	7 µg

If there is any doubt about the vitamin status of a baby under six months, for example infants breast fed by a mother in poor vitamin status, vitamin drops can be given from one month.

Infants living in areas where the water is not fluoridated should receive fluoride supplements (see page 147).

Eating for future health

Relative to their size, babies and young children have high requirements for energy and nutrients. Their capacity for food is smaller than that of adults, so the foods they eat should provide energy and nutrients in a compact form. High fibre/low fat diets recommended for adults (see Part 1, page 5) are therefore not suitable for children under two years of age, as foods which feature in such diets can be low in energy, bulky and filling. However, between the ages of two and five most children should be able to progress towards eating a diet relatively low in fat and high in fibre, as recommended for adults.

The need for young children to be established on a diet containing nutrient-dense foods is emphasized by a survey of disadvantaged families in Glamorgan (Barker, 1987). A report by Pugliese and colleagues (1987) showed that children diagnosed as failing to thrive but showing no signs of illness were being fed low calorie, low fat diets, which were often free of snacks, by parents concerned about future risk of heart disease or obesity (see page 41). Once appropriate dietary advice was acted upon, the children began to grow again. It is important, therefore, to balance the need for advice on a diet which will benefit future health with that which will ensure proper growth and development.

The taste for sugar and salt can be established early in life, with well-established negative consequences. High intakes of sugar contribute to the development of dental caries (see page 146) and possibly to obesity.

The sodium which is naturally present in milk and weaning foods will meet requirements. Additional salt is not needed. In adults, high salt intakes are a causal factor in the development of hypertension. The use of salt should, therefore, be discouraged in young children in order to promote a preference for less salt in adulthood. In particular, data exist to suggest that adults with high blood pressure often had raised blood pressure in childhood (Schachter et al., 1982). Korner et al. (1985) describe high blood pressure as a self-perpetuating disorder, the origins of which can lie in very early childhood. Consequently primary prevention should begin early in life (Culpepper et al., 1983).

Extra sugar and salt should therefore not be added to babies' food (see Table 2.4).

References

Barker W (1987) Child development project. In *National Dairy Council Fact File 2. Nutrition and Children Aged One to Five*. London, National Dairy Council.

Buttriss JL and Gray J (1995) *The Nutrition of Infants and Preschool Children. Fact File 2 (revised)*. London, National Dairy Council.

Cole TJ (1993) The use and construction of anthropometric growth reference standards. *Nutrition Research Reviews* **6**, 19–50.

Cole TJ (1994) Do growth chart centiles need a face lift? *British Medical Journal* **308**, 641–2.

Culpepper WS et al. (1983) Cardiac status in juvenile borderline hypertension. *Annals of Internal Medicine* **98**, 1–7.

Dallman PR (1986) Iron deficiency in weaning: a nutritional problem on the way to resolution. *Acta Paediatrica* (Suppl) **323**, 59–67.

Department of Health, Committee on Medical Aspects of Food Policy (1991) *Dietary Reference Values for Food Energy and Nutrients for the United Kingdom. Report on Health and Social Subjects 41*. London, HMSO.

Department of Health, Committee on Medical Aspects of Food Policy (1994) *Weaning and the Weaning Diet. Report on Health and Social Subjects 45*. London, HMSO.

Department of Health and Social Security (1980) *Artificial Feeds for the Young Infant. Report on Health and Social Subjects 18*. London, HMSO.

Department of Health and Social Security, Committee on Medical Aspects of Food Policy (1988) *Present Day Practice in Infant Feeding: Third Report*. London, HMSO.

Eastham EJ et al. (1982) Antigenicity of infant formulas and the induction of systemic immunological tolerance by oral feeding: cows' milk and soya milk. *Journal of Pediatric Gastroenterological Nutrition* **1**, 23–28.

EEC (1991) Commission Directive on infant formulae and follow-on formulae. *Official Journal of the European Communities* **L175**, 35–49.

ESPGAN Committee on Nutrition (1977) Guidelines on infant nutrition. I Recommendations for the composition of an adapted formula. *Acta Paediatrica Scandinavica* (Suppl) **262**, 1–20.

ESPGAN Committee on Nutrition (1981) Guidelines on infant nutrition. II Recommendations for the composition of follow-up formula and beikost. *Acta Paediatrica Scandinavica* (Suppl) **287**.

ESPGAN Committee on Nutrition (1987) Nutrition and feeding of pre-term infants. *Acta Paediatrica Scandinavica* (Suppl) **336**.

Fairweather-Tait SJ (1992) Iron deficiency in infancy: easy to prevent — or is it? *European Journal of Clinical Nutrition* **46**, Suppl. 4, S9–14.

Farquharson J et al. (1992) Infant cerebral cortex phospholipid fatty acid composition and diet. *Lancet* **340**, 810–13.

Freeman JV et al. (1995) Cross sectional stature and weight reference curves for the UK 1990. *Archives of Disease in Childhood* **73**, 17–24.

Howie PW et al. (1990) Protective effect of breast feeding against infection. *British Medical Journal* **300**, 11–16.

Idjradinata P et al. (1994) Adverse effects of iron supplementation on weight gain of iron-replete young children. *Lancet* **343**, 1252–4.

Korner PI et al. (1985) Role of cardiac and vascular amplifiers in the maintenance of hypertension and the effect of reversal of cardiovascular hypertrophy. *Clinical and Experimental Pharmacology and Physiology* **12**, 205–9.

Lawson M (1992) Baby formulas. *Community Outlook*, August, pp 23–29.

Lucas A et al. (1992) Breast milk and subsequent intelligence quotient in children born preterm. *Lancet* **339**, 261–4.

Martin J (1978) *Infant Feeding 1975: Attitudes and Practice in England and Wales*. Office of Population Censuses and Surveys. London, HMSO.

Martin J and Monk J (1982) *Infant Feeding 1980*. Office of Population Censuses and Surveys. London, HMSO.

Martin J and White A (1988) *Infant Feeding in 1985*. Office of Population Censuses and Surveys. London, HMSO.

Mills A and Tyler H (1992) *Food and Nutrient Intakes of British Infants aged 6–12 Months*. Ministry of Agriculture, Fisheries and Food. London, HMSO.

National Nutrition Council (Norway) (1993) Nutrition policy objectives and measures: food and nutrition. In *Challenges in Health Promotion and Prevention*. Report of the Sorting Number 37, 1992–93. Ch. 11.

Oski FA and Landow SA (1980) Inhibition of iron absorption from human milk by baby food. *American Journal of Disease in Childhood* **134**, 459–60.

Pugliese MT et al. (1987) Parental health beliefs as a cause of failure to thrive. *Pediatrics* **80,** 175–82.

Rennie JJ (1988) *Food Intolerance. Layman's Guide No. 26.* Leatherhead Food Research Association.

Royal College of Physicians and British Nutrition Foundation (1984) Food intolerance and food aversion. *Journal of the Royal College of Physicians* **18,** 1–41.

Royal College of Midwives (1991) *Successful Breast-feeding.* 2nd edn. London, Churchill Livingstone.

Schachter J et al. (1982) Blood pressure during the first two years of life. *American Journal of Epidemiology* **116,** 29–41.

Taitz LS and Scholey E (1989) Are babies more satisfied by casein-based formulas? *Archives of Diseases in Childhood* **64,** 619–21.

Walter T (1993) Impact of iron deficiency on cognition in infancy and childhood. *European Journal of Clinical Nutrition* **47,** 307–16.

White A et al. (1992) *Infant Feeding 1990.* Office of Population Censuses and Surveys. London, HMSO.

Further reading

Buttriss J and Hyman K (Eds) (1994) *Children in Focus.* Proceedings of a Conference, 1993. London, National Dairy Council.

Buttriss J and Hyman K (Eds) (1995) *The Growing Cycle: Child, Mother, Child.* Proceedings of a conference, 1994. London, National Dairy Council.

3

Preschool children

Key points

1. Children aged one to five have relatively high nutrient needs in comparison with their size and the quantity of food sometimes consumed by this age group. The quality (nutrient density) of their diet is therefore very important.

2. From a behavioural point of view, and given that societal changes mean that families increasingly do not eat meals as a family unit, snacking can be a usual feature of the preschool diet. Provided the snacks are nourishing, this need not be a problem. But the provision of sugary, relatively low nutrient snack foods such as sweets and biscuits, should be limited to infrequent occasions and teeth should be brushed afterwards. This is particularly important from the dental health point of view.

3. The transition from the infant diet to that recommended for adults, rich in starch and fibre but low in fat, should occur gradually. A low fat, high fibre diet can be very bulky, and too rapid a change can result in young children feeling full before they have eaten enough to satisfy nutrient needs.

4. The principles of a balanced diet, incorporating nutrient-rich foods selected from the four main food groups, applies to this group.

5. Cows' milk is usually an important part of the diet for this age group. Children under two should have whole milk but after this age semi-skimmed milk is suitable provided the child's overall food and energy intake is satisfactory.

6. Erratic eating patterns may occur in this age group and it may take time to steer children towards adult meal patterns.

7. Faddy eating is common but a healthy child is unlikely to starve himself. The cause of faddiness should be established where possible and parents should be warned that overt concern may exacerbate the problem.

8. Advice to parents should emphasize the need for inclusion of sources of iron to reduce the risk of anaemia.

9. Where constipation occurs parents may need advice on the inclusion of adequate amounts of fibre-rich foods in their child's diet.

10. Toddler diarrhoea is common and parents may need reassurance.

Food and nutrient intake in preschool children

The term 'preschool children' is used to define children aged one to five. Children in this age group have relatively high nutrient needs in relation to the amount of food they are sometimes prepared to eat, they undergo quite rapid growth and development, and they are usually physically active. Hence the quality or nutrient density of their diets is of particular importance. Contrary to popular belief, the energy cost of growth in children aged one to five years is less than 1% of their total energy requirement and nutritional needs (per kilogram body weight) are not as high as in infancy (Stordy, 1995). Nevertheless, if food intake is inadequate, an early sign will be a faltering in growth. But of course, young children have a limited capacity for eating large quantities of food, are often too 'busy' to eat, or cannot be bothered, and so they generally require relatively small meals as well as suitable between-meal snacks of good nutrient density. A nutrient-dense diet is one comprising foods rich in essential nutrients, whereas an energy-dense one comprises foods which are concentrated sources of energy but which do not necessarily also provide essential nutrients.

The eating patterns of preschool children can be erratic too, and at times the range of foods they are prepared to eat can be limited. This is often a source of great concern for parents, who need to be reassured that the child's weight may remain static for a week or two and that weight gain is variable. They should be encouraged not to pay too much attention to weekly fluctuations but should expect their child to gain weight over a period of, say, three months.

For information on suitable growth standards, see section on Infant Feeding and Weaning, page 22.

Establishing good dietary patterns

Developing good appetite control is important. If a child drinks copious amounts of juice between meals or is allowed to snack on foods of poor nutrient density such as sweets and packet snack foods, it is not surprising that he or she will have little appetite at mealtimes. If main course foods are refused, the child should not be offered sweets or biscuits as an alternative.

It is recognized that establishing appropriate eating habits in young children is important from both nutritional and developmental points of view (DH, 1994). Preferences established in childhood for example for sugary, fatty or salty foods may have an impact both on adult eating habits and adult health.

The diet of young infants (for example, breast milk) contains about 54% of energy from fat, no fibre, and simple sugars rather than starch. This is clearly quite different from the adult dietary recommendations — 35% of food energy from fat, 11% from sugars, plenty of starch and plenty of non-starch polysaccharides (fibre) (18 g/day) (see Part 1, page 5). Yet a transition needs to be made from one to the other, during early childhood.

The preschool years should be seen as a time when this transition is made. The rate and extent to which this can be achieved in this age group will depend on the appetite of the individual child. Although a diet meeting adult guidelines is likely to be bulky for the under-twos, most children over two can manage a diet with a reduced fat content and containing foods rich in fibre and starch (DH, 1994).

However, doubt has been expressed about whether current dietary guidelines, aimed at the prevention of adult disorders, are appropriate for preschool children (for example, Stordy, 1995). Most parents are sensible about the amount of fibre they give to young children. But a diet which is unduly bulky may satisfy the appetite but not the requirement for energy and nutrients (Pugliese et al., 1987; Nicklas et al., 1992).

Consequently, on occasions malnourished children will be encountered for whom the energy density of the diet needs to be increased. The overall quality of the diet, that is the nutrient density, may also need attention.

Quality of preschool diets

Personal observation reveals that many children, including preschool children, eat a less than balanced diet, containing many sweets, biscuits, fizzy drinks and packet snack foods high in fat and salt. In such diets, too great a proportion of energy is derived from fat, sugar or both, and there is insufficient starch and fibre. Intakes of specific vitamins and minerals may also be poor.

A survey of the nutritional intake and status of children aged $1^1/_2$–$4^1/_2$ years (Gregory et al., 1995), undertaken as part of the National Diet and Nutrition Survey, was published in early 1995. This survey provides detailed information about the diets of such children and whether these support a good nutritional status. A detailed summary of the key findings can be found in Buttriss and Gray (1995). However, in general terms the survey indicated that it is the quality of the diet rather than the quantity of food eaten that provides cause for concern.

The survey revealed that preschool children today are taller than they were 27 years ago when the last survey was conducted, but 1 in 12 of this age group is anaemic (see page 44), 17% have active tooth decay (see page 43) and, on the whole, preschool children are eating large amounts of salt and sugar, and insufficient fruit and vegetables.

This national study and a small study of 153 preschool children in Edinburgh carried out between 1988 and 1990 both reported that the mean energy intake of the children was below the estimated average requirement for this age group (Payne and Belton, 1992a; 1992b). However anthropometric measurements indicated that growth was normal, and the values are within the limits of the range of estimates for total energy expenditure of two and three year olds using the doubly labelled water technique (Prentice et al., 1988; Davies et al., 1991).

Children with higher energy intakes tended to have higher NSP (fibre) intakes. Average intakes of total sugars were high (about 30% of total energy) relative to intakes of starch. In common with other studies (see DH, 1989), there was a marked reciprocal relationship between fat and sugar intake. In older children, it has been observed that sugar intake is lower but at the expense of fat intake (Nelson, 1991; McNeill et al., 1991). In both the national study and that by Payne and Belton, much of the intake of sugars was supplied by soft drinks and fruit juice. As fat and sugar are the two major providers of energy, a balance needs to be struck in the provision of foods containing these.

The mean fat intakes of the children in both surveys were in the region of 34%–36% of dietary energy and thus within the range suggested for older children and adults (DH, 1991). However, the COMA report on weaning (DH, 1994) states clearly that full implementation of a fat-restricted diet is inappropriate for children under the age of five.

As long as growth is maintained, there is probably no need to be concerned about energy intake of children, although dietary quality should be considered too.

Calcium intakes were generally good (because most of the children consumed milk regularly) but average iron intakes were low and almost a quarter of the $1^1/_2$–$2^1/_2$ year olds had iron intakes below the lower reference nutrient intake (Gregory et al., 1995). In both studies, the vitamin and mineral intakes of the children varied widely, but a minority were found to have low intakes of vitamins A, C and D, and zinc.

Vitamin and mineral status tended to be worse in children from poorer families (see Chapter 8).

As with other age groups, a balanced diet can be achieved by offering a wide range of foods selected from the four groups which each contain nutrient-rich foods (see Appendix 1 and Part 1, page 31). Although serving sizes will inevitably be small, the ratio of servings from the four groups still applies — at least four daily servings from cereals, and from fruit and vegetables, three servings of milk and milk products, and two servings of meat and meat alternatives.

Cows' milk will be an important item in the diet of most children in this age group. The recommendation that they receive a minimum of 350 ml a day will ensure that calcium intake is adequate, and will make substantial contributions to the requirements for other nutrients. The Department of Health (1994) recommends whole milk as the main type of milk for the under-fives, although it is acknowledged that once a child is eating a wide range of foods, then the energy content of the milk becomes less important. Therefore, beyond the age of two years, provided a child is eating well, semi-skimmed milk is acceptable. Skimmed milk is not recommended as the main type of milk used before the age of five years because it contains no vitamin A and has a much lower energy content (DH, 1994).

Vitamin drops containing vitamins A, C and D are recommended by the Department of

Health (1994) for preschool children preferably until age five. Supplementation with these important vitamins acts as an 'insurance policy' during the transition from milk to a mixed diet, once infant formula is stopped.

Snacking versus small frequent meals

Consumption of small frequent meals is often a main feature of the diets of preschool children, particularly for those with a limited capacity for food. Although this mode of eating is quite acceptable, it is important to distinguish between snack meals comprising nutritious foods and snacks of poor nutritional quality, high in fat, sugar and salt.

Snacks should be seen as a means of contributing to total nutrient needs rather than merely satisfying hunger and the desire to eat. Inappropriate snacks between meals may satisfy a child's appetite and therefore suppress the desire to eat more nutritious foods at normal mealtimes. Children with poor appetites or those who are often hungry between meals may fare better on five nutritious mini-meals rather than three meals and two nutritionally poor between-meal snacks.

Foods which are rich in fat and/or sugar, but of relatively low nutrient density, for example confectionery and biscuits, can readily satisfy hunger and suppress appetite in a young child. Frequent consumption of sugary snacks and drinks can also damage developing teeth (see Chapter 13).

Parents should therefore be advised to limit considerably the provision of high fat, sugary and salty snacks, particularly in the early preschool years. Rather than giving them between meals, such foods could be included as an addition to a meal based on nutrient-dense foods, for example at tea time.

Snacks considered more suitable include:

- fruit and pieces of raw vegetable (e.g. celery, carrots)
- bread, breadsticks, crispbreads, sandwiches made with a small amount of jam, pâté or meat/fish paste, cheese (especially lower fat varieties), tuna, sardines, lean meat, egg
- a drink of milk and a plain biscuit
- yogurt or fromage frais
- low sugar breakfast cereal (dry or with milk)
- a bun or scone
- a small piece of cheese
- plain popcorn (e.g. made in a microwave) rather than crisps.

Water or milk are advised as the most suitable drinks for children (DH, 1994), and drinks such as fruit juice or squash should be dilute, restricted to meal times and never consumed in a feeding bottle or at bedtime. This advice, important from a dental health point of view, is supported by data from a dental survey of $1^{1}/_{2}$–$4^{1}/_{2}$ year olds (Hinds and Gregory, 1995). For example, dental decay was far more common in those children who took drinks of squash or juice to bed than among those who had water or milk.

Child immunization at one year of age provides an opportunity to talk to mothers (or other carers) about children's diets. The child's development and behaviour could also be discussed at this time, and the occasion could offer an opportunity for nurses to develop a check-list for use as an audit tool.

Parents may appreciate ideas on how to deal with requests for snacks such as sweets and biscuits. Banning sweets altogether usually does not work. Other ideas include:

- keeping sweets and chocolates for the end of mealtimes only
- making sure children brush their teeth after eating sweets and other sweet foods
- allowing sweets only on certain days of the week
- explaining why they cannot have sweets every day and letting them help decide the best way of cutting down
- thinking of other treats and asking relatives and friends to do the same; badges, stickers, colouring books, crayons and hair slides may be a bit more expensive but they do last longer.

Common diet-related problems

Faddy eating

Faddy eating is common among preschool children and is a normal developmental stage, indicating that the child is growing up and asserting his or her independence. It normally passes once the child is at school and becomes aware of the importance of 'conforming' with his/her peers. Although some children at this age seem hardly to eat a thing, healthy children are very unlikely to starve themselves (Birch et al., 1991) and so parents should be encouraged to avoid making an issue of this pattern of eating.

Parents can be reassured that no individual food is essential, although they should try to encourage children to eat as wide a variety of foods as possible — even if only in very small amounts. They should be warned against allowing the consumption of foods such as cakes, biscuits, savoury packet snack foods, sweets and sugary drinks to become substitutes for other foods. Reinforcement of this sort of inappropriate eating habit can lead to poor eating patterns throughout childhood and in later life (see page 41).

It is also important to establish the reason for the faddiness. Is it genuine poor appetite or is the child eating too much between meals? Young children with so-called poor appetites are often found to be drinking large volumes of juice, sugary drinks (Hourihane and Rolles, 1995) or milk between meals, which limits their capacity for food at mealtimes. Another factor is prolonged bottle feeding, which has implications for dental health because of the way that the milk or juice bathes the teeth when sucked through a bottle, or even from a feeder-beaker. Use of feeding bottles, particularly for squash and juice, is not recommended after one year of age (DH, 1994).

While up to a pint of milk a day can be provided with benefit, children with a poor appetite should be offered water if they are thirsty **between** meals, rather than juice or soft drinks. The presentation of food can also be highly relevant. The temperature of the food, the quantity provided and whether or not it is adequately chopped, can easily put a child off eating.

Another important factor is the environment in which the food is eaten. It should be quiet and peaceful and the child should receive the full attention of the carer. This is particularly important for young children, who may need a lot of help. Appropriate attention from the carer can be an important factor in preventing feeding problems.

Some children will not eat if there are lots of distractions around them, including the television. However, in some cases children who are restless at mealtimes will sit at the table and eat, rather than run around, if they have a focus such as the television.

Emphasizing the importance of the eating occasion and its social implications by sitting at the table and eating as a family may help. Faddy eating may also respond positively to involvement in the preparation of the meal or in laying the table. If the faddiness is simply a means of getting attention, parents might try ignoring the child when he or she refuses to eat, but giving praise and attention when a mouthful is eaten. Food refusal is also often a means of seeking attention.

Anaemia and low iron intake

In recent years, there has been a number of reports of low iron status and iron deficiency anaemia among infants and preschool children (Aukett et al., 1986; James et al., 1989; Marder et al., 1990; Mills, 1990; Gregory et al., 1995). Low iron status seems particularly prevalent among immigrant children (Illingworth, 1986; Duggan et al., 1992), and those living in families with low income (see Chapter 13 and Part 3, Anaemia in Children and Adults). Children for whom a poor weaning diet, low in iron, has been coupled with unmodified cows' milk early in infancy seem particularly vulnerable. Unmodified cows' milk provides a wide range of essential nutrients and is particularly important for calcium, but is a poor source of iron.

Provided infants and preschool children are given a wide variety of nutrient-rich foods including some rich in iron, inadequate iron intake is unlikely. Red meat, liver (and liver pâté) and kidneys are important sources of well-absorbed iron. Other useful sources include chicken, low fat sausages and burgers, oily fish such as sardines, fortified breakfast cereals, eggs, baked beans, bread, dried apricots, lentils and dark green vegetables such as broccoli (see page 34 for more details). Chocolate provides some iron and can be a significant source of iron for children whose diets are very poor; nevertheless parents should not be encouraged to give chocolate to their children.

Iron from non-meat sources is less well absorbed and mothers should be encouraged to provide a source of vitamin C, for example fruit, vegetables or diluted pure fruit juice at meals, as this will aid the absorption of iron from foods eaten at the same meal.

There are a number of other promotors and inhibitors of iron absorption. These are discussed in detail in Part 1 (page 29) and in Part 3, Anaemia in Adults and Children. One such inhibitor is tannin in tea. Children who are poor eaters and so whose iron intake may be low should not be given tea at mealtimes as this may prevent absorption of iron taken at the same meal. Although iron is to be found in green vegetables, it is often poorly absorbed because of the oxalate to which it is bound.

Where it is difficult to guarantee that the diet will contain adequate iron, formula milk or follow-on milk can be used as a safeguard over the age of one year. But this cannot realistically be a long-term measure and the diet should still be improved gradually, because establishment of good eating patterns during early childhood is very important for future health.

Constipation

Constipation is quite a common problem in children (Clayden, 1989). The bowel habits of breast and bottle-fed infants are quite different but transfer from either of these to a mixed diet can cause temporary constipation or loose stools. During weaning there should be a gradual progression from the fibre-free diet of the infant to a diet containing fibre from a variety of sources: cereals, pulses, vegetables and fruit (see Part 1, page 33). Although before the age of one it is not advisable to introduce too bulky a diet, once appetite increases there is no reason why wholegrain cereal foods (not bran supplemented) should not be introduced. If fibre-rich foods are not introduced into the diet in adequate amounts, then constipation may become a problem. However, constipation may also result from an inadequate fluid intake or be associated with a reluctance to empty the bowel; the latter may necessitate advice on behaviour modification. It may also be associated with an anal fissure where a paediatric opinion may be required.

When constipation occurs, dietary advice should be given. It should be possible to alleviate it by an increased consumption of fruit, vegetables, pulses and of cereal products such as bread and high-fibre breakfast cereals, and by an increase in fluid intake, particularly water or diluted fruit juices.

Some severely constipated children have overflow diarrhoea. This should be distinguished from normal diarrhoea and treated accordingly.

Toddler diarrhoea

Toddler diarrhoea, seen at the age of about 18 months, is a common phenomenon of unknown cause. The stools contain identifiable items of undigested food, particularly vegetables. The main course of action is to reassure parents that the condition is common, not serious, will pass and that undigested vegetables in the stools are fairly normal in young children (Carne, 1988, 1991). In addition, large amounts of sugary drinks should be discouraged as these seem to make matters worse. In deciding on the management, it is important to establish what the parent means by 'diarrhoea', how long the condition has persisted, whether it has happened before, and whether other family members have the same problem. It is also important to assess whether a normal growth pattern is occurring by weighing the child at intervals. If weight gain is normal, there is usually less need for concern.

In mild cases, it is debatable whether there is any significant fluid or electrolyte loss but a simple sugar or glucose solution (perhaps with a few grains of salt) can be beneficial (Carne, 1988). This 'clear fluid' regimen should continue for about 24 hours, after which solids can gradually be introduced, for example dry toast smeared with a little jam (no butter or margarine). In most cases, recovery will be complete in 48–72 hours. In more severe cases, dehydration needs careful management, the basic principles being to replace fluid and electrolytes. But most children with diarrhoea are at little or no risk of dehydration. There is usually no need for antibiotic treatment (Carne, 1988).

Chronic diarrhoea is a different problem and needs a thorough investigation to exclude diagnoses such as coeliac disease, lactose malabsorption and milk protein allergy (see relevant sections in Part 3).

References

Auckett MA et al. (1986) Treatment with iron increases weight gain and psychomotor development. *Archives of Disease in Childhood* **61**, 849–57.

Birch LL et al. (1991) The variability of young children's energy intake. *New England Journal of Medicine* **324**, 323–5.

Buttriss JL and Gray J (1995) *The Nutrition of Infants and Preschool Children. Fact File 2 (revised)*. London, National Dairy Council.

Carne S (1988) A no-nonsense approach to diarrhoea. *Mims Magazine*, November, 73–76.

Carne S (1991) Diarrhoea. *Maternal and Child Health*. April, 112–4.

Clayden GS (1989) Constipation in childhood. *British Medical Journal* **299**, 1116–7.

Davies PSW et al. (1991) Total energy expenditure during childhood and adolescence. *Proceedings of the Nutrition Society* **50**, 14A.

Department of Health (1989) *Dietary Sugars and Human Disease*. London, HMSO.

Department of Health, Committee on Medical Aspects of Food Policy (1991) *Dietary Reference Values for Food Energy and Nutrients for the United Kingdom. Report on Health and Social Subjects 41*. London, HMSO.

Department of Health, Committee on Medical Aspects of Food Policy (1994) *Weaning and the Weaning Diet. Report on Health and Social Subjects 45*. London, HMSO.

Duggan MB et al. (1992) The weaning diet of healthy Asian children living in Sheffield. *Journal of Human Nutrition and Dietetics* **5**, 189–200.

Gregory JR et al. (1995) *National Diet and Nutrition Survey of Children aged $1^1/_2$–$4^1/_2$ Years*. London, HMSO.

Hinds K and Gregory JR (1995) *National Diet and Nutrition Survey of Children aged $1^1/_2$–$4^1/_2$ Years. Volume 2: Report of the Dental Survey*. London, HMSO.

Hourihane J O'B and Rolles CJ (1995) Morbidity from excessive intake of high energy fluids: the 'squash drinking syndrome'. *Archives of Disease in Childhood* **72**, 141–3.

Illingworth RS (1986) Anaemia and child health surveillance. *Archives of Disease in Childhood* **61**, 1151–2.

James J et al. (1989) Preventing iron deficiency in preschool children by implementing educational and screening programme in an inner city practice. *British Medical Journal* **299**, 838–40.

Marder E et al. (1990) Discovering anaemia at child health clinics. *Archives of Disease in Childhood* **65**, 892–4.

McNeill G et al. (1991) Nutrient intake in school children: some practical considerations. *Proceedings of the Nutrition Society* **50**, 37–43.

Mills AF (1990) Surveillance for anaemia: risk factors in patterns of mild intake. *Archives of Disease in Childhood* **65**, 428–31.

Nelson M (1991) Food, vitamins and IQ. *Proceedings of the Nutrition Society* **50**, 29–35.

Nicklas TA et al. (1992) Nutrient adequacy of low fat intakes for children: the Bogalusa Heart Study. *Pediatrics* **89**, 221–8.

Payne JA and Belton NR (1992a) Nutrient intake and growth in pre-school children, I. Comparison of energy intake and sources of energy with growth. *Journal of Human Nutrition and Dietetics* **5**, 287–98.

Payne JA and Belton NR (1992b) Nutrient intake and growth in pre-school children II. Intake of minerals and vitamins. *Journal of Human Nutrition and Dietetics* **5**, 299–304.

Prentice AM et al. (1988) Are current dietary guidelines for young children a prescription for overfeeding? *Lancet* **2**, 1066–9.

Pugliese T et al. (1987) Parental health beliefs as a cause of failure to thrive. *Paediatrics* **80**, 175–82.

Stordy BJ (1995) Is it appropriate to apply adult healthy eating guidelines to babies and young children? In Buttriss JL and Hyman K (Eds) *The Growing Cycle: Child, Mother, Child*. Proceedings of a conference, 1994. London, National Dairy Council.

4

Schoolchildren

Key points

1. Children's diets should meet nutrient and energy needs, promote health and be enjoyable. The basic principles of nutrition outlined in Part 1 apply.

2. The importance of establishing good eating patterns should be emphasized, as this is likely to influence eating behaviour in adult life.

3. There is evidence that the diets of the majority of children are imbalanced, providing excessive amounts of foods rich in fat and sugar relative to foods rich in complex carbohydrates. This may have serious implications for the future health of these children. In general, children's intake of vitamins and minerals is adequate but there is evidence that intakes of iron and calcium, in particular, may be low in some children.

4. Dental caries has its peak prevalence during childhood and can be reduced by avoiding the almost continuous consumption of foods and drinks during the day which occurs with some children, and specifically by a decrease in the quantity and frequency of sugar consumption. In this context, advice on appropriate snacks and drinks is important.

5. Older children, especially girls, who eat outside school at lunch-time, may be at particular risk of poor intakes of iron, calcium and riboflavin. There is therefore a risk of anaemia in these girls, specially in those who adopt a vegetarian style of eating. Future bone health may also be threatened.

6. The main nutritional problem among children is not malnutrition but overweight. The best way to prevent overweight and obsession with body image is to discourage high fat and high sugar foods, and to encourage exercise. Activity levels among some children, particularly some girls, are very low.

7. Children who are overweight, especially after the age of 11 years, may carry their problems into adult life, and therefore require treatment to prevent the progression of overweight to a more serious degree of obesity. Severe obesity and eating disorders such as anorexia and bulimia nervosa require specialist advice. Ideally, overweight should be prevented in the first place by promoting a more active lifestyle and an energy intake which matches needs.

Children's diets should sustain growth, promote health and be enjoyable. The demands for some nutrients, for example calcium, increase substantially during the pubertal growth spurt of adolescence (see Part 1, Appendix 1), and proportionately, that is per kg body weight, children require a greater nutrient intake than adults. Hence the **nutrient density** of the food eaten — the nutrient content relative to the energy content — should be high.

There is a growing concern that the unbalanced nature of the diets of some children (see below) together with the low levels of physical activity among children (Armstrong et al., 1990; Balding, 1995; Fox, 1994), particularly girls, could have an extremely detrimental effect on their health in later life.

The food consumed in childhood, particularly in adolescence, can set the pattern for future food preferences and eating behaviour in adult life. This in turn can influence long-term health, for example contributing to the development of dental caries, obesity, non-insulin dependent diabetes, cardio-vascular disease, bowel problems and osteo-porosis.

As children grow older, their food choices may be influenced increasingly by external factors such as friends and media-led fashions. Emotional factors and attitudes to appearance and body image also become important, especially in girls. Erratic eating patterns and faddy eating are common in adolescence.

Food and nutrient intake

The most recent national survey of school-children's eating habits was conducted in 1983 (DHSS, 1989). It indicated that the diets of some children comprise a high pro-portion of snack foods, rich in both fat and sugar, and sugary soft drinks (see below). Although these data are now 10 years old, they have been supported by the findings of several recent, though far smaller, studies (see page 49).

The DHSS (1989) survey concerned child-ren aged 10–11 and 14–15 years. There was concern that the diets of many children were unbalanced, containing too much fat and too few foods rich in starch and fibre. For the four age-sex groups, energy intake from fat ranged between 37% and 39% of energy. Three-quarters of the children had fat intakes above 35% of energy (the recommended target level; DH, 1991), and about one-fifth of the boys and one-third of the girls had intakes of fat providing more than 40% of dietary energy. The fact that some children were overweight was also of concern.

In the original analysis of the data, in relation to the dietary standards (recommended daily amounts — RDAs — at the time of the study), there was evidence of low intakes of iron and calcium among some of the children. Since the data were published, new dietary reference values (DRVs) have been published (DH, 1991), and reference nutrient intakes (RNIs), equivalent to the old RDAs, have been increased in this age group for both calcium and iron, nutrients which were marginal in the diets of some of the children.

When intakes of the children are compared with these new values, the iron intake of over a third of 10–11 year old girls and about one-third of 14–15 year old girls falls below the lower reference nutrient intake (LRNI). This is the level below which almost everybody is likely to be deficient and so these girls were at high risk of iron deficiency, especially if men-strual losses were heavy (see also page 50, and Part 1, Appendix 2 for foods rich in iron).

Average intakes of calcium in the DHSS study were considerably below the 1991 reference nutrient intake of 1000 mg per day for boys and 800 mg per day for girls of this age group (the amounts judged to meet or exceed the needs of virtually all children of this age). The average intakes for each age and sex group hide a wide distribution of intakes and there were some children, parti-cularly older girls, who were consuming less than 300 mg of calcium each day because of a low consumption of milk, bread and cereals. Almost 20% of the girls had intakes which were unlikely to be adequate in that they were below the lower reference nutrient intake of 450 mg/day. Such low intake, if habitual, could jeopardize achievement of peak bone mass, which could in turn have implications for future bone health.

The results of several smaller, but more recent surveys have confirmed these findings. In studies of 143 children aged 11–12 years (Nelson, 1991) and 405 children of the same age (Rugg-Gunn et al., 1991) there was evidence that children were selecting diets which did not conform to current recom-mendations on complex carbohydrates, fat and extrinsic sugars. Diets were also low in fruit and vegetables, and in iron and calcium.

A review by the Caroline Walker Trust (1992) of these and other recent studies concerning children's diets has drawn the following conclusions:

- Children's diets are high in fat and the proportion of energy derived from fat has not fallen in recent years.

- Consumption of 'added' sugar is high and has not fallen in recent years.

- Intake of fibre in general, and fruit and vegetables in particular, is low and reflects adult social class and regional variations.

- Intakes of iron are low, particularly among adolescent girls.

- Calcium intakes are also relatively low.

- Folate intakes appear to be low.

- Low energy intakes, related to slimming, are common among teenagers and in such individuals low intakes of calcium, iron, and vitamins A, B_2 and B_6 are particularly likely.

- Children living in low income families sometimes have particularly low intakes of several nutrients, for example vitamins C and A. Also, the overall nutrient intake of these children depends more on school meals than does that of children from wealthier backgrounds.

School meals

Before the Education Act of 1980, nutritional standards for school meals were set by the Department of Education and Science. School meals were then expected to provide one-third of a child's daily requirement of protein, energy and some vitamins and minerals. Now, the local education authorities are obliged only to provide a place for children to eat packed lunches brought to school. In 1988, changes to the system of benefits resulted in some children's entitlement to free school meals being replaced by direct cash payments to the family — which may or may not be spent on food.

In England in 1991, 42% of schoolchildren had school meals, and a little over a quarter of these received free meals. Schoolchildren qualify for school meals if parents provide evidence that they are in receipt of Income Support. Children whose parents receive Income Support are also entitled to free school milk (at midday). Local education authorities lost the power to provide free milk to other pupils in 1986. Families receiving Family Credit get a cash payment instead.

The provision of food at school for many children, especially the older ones, is now in the form of a cash-cafeteria service. There is therefore little control over the choice of foods a child makes.

The DHSS (1989) survey showed that older children especially the girls, who were eating out of school in take-away, café or 'fast food' outlets were selecting foods of rather low nutrient density. They had a lower intake of many nutrients, especially iron but also calcium and vitamin A.

The pattern of snacking and meal skipping was also evident in a survey of the eating habits of teenagers and young adults (15–25 year olds) in the UK (Bull, 1985). Breakfast was omitted by 18% of those surveyed and girls were more likely to miss this meal.

Balding and colleagues have routinely been collecting information on eating habits in children aged 12–16 years since 1981. The 1991 sample included almost 24 000 pupils from a total of 142 schools across the UK and included questions on school meals (Balding, 1992). In general, more boys than girls ate in the school cafeteria and the proportion fell with increasing age of the child. A similar trend with age was seen in the proportion taking packed lunches, though these tended to be favoured more by girls. There were also significant increases in the number of older pupils eating take-aways at lunch-time or purportedly going home for lunch. Together these accounted for about 40% of the lunch-time eating habits of 15–16 year olds. Worryingly, 11% of girls aged 14–16 years and 5% of boys said they had no lunch.

There is a need to target children in schools, but also parents, so that eating both within the school and within the family context can reflect current nutritional guidelines. A Health of the Nation project team is developing voluntary nutritional guidance for school food providers.

Ideas for packed lunches

A useful guide for a nutritionally balanced packed lunch, based on the food groups discussed in Appendix 1 and Part 1 (page 31) is that it provides at least one item from each of the bread/cereals group and the fruit/vegetables group, an item from the meat/alternatives group, and an item from the milk/milk products group. Below are some examples:

- **Cereal group serving:** bread as a sandwich, a pitta bread (with filling), a chapatti, a low sugar scone, a currant bun, rice or pasta salad

- **Fruit/vegetable serving:** apple or other fruit, a tomato, sticks of raw vegetables, such as carrots, salad — either as part of the sandwich or separately, a carton of unsweetened fruit juice

- **Milk serving:** small carton of milk, pot of yogurt, cheese as sandwich filling, a small lump of cheese

- **Meat and alternatives group serving:** lean meat, tinned fish, egg or peanut butter as sandwich filling, hard boiled egg, portion of dahl.

Only when foods from each of the four groups have been included should additional foods such as biscuits or crisps be considered. The latter may have a part to play in the lunch-boxes of those children with larger appetites, but they should not be the main components of the lunch.

Examples of three lunch-boxes:

- Sandwich of wholemeal bread, lean ham, sliced tomato
  Carrot and celery sticks
  A yogurt
  A carton of unsweetened fruit juice
  A slice of fruit cake

- A pitta bread filled with chicken and salad
  A tomato
  A satsuma
  2 oatcakes and a cube of cheese

- Hard-boiled egg
  Chunk of French bread
  Small packet of unsalted nuts and raisins
  Small carton of UHT milk/milk shake
  An orange.

Implications of changing eating habits

Some children, especially those aged 11 years and above, are selecting diets from a range of snack foods rather than meals put together in a 'traditional' way. Although such diets can meet the requirements for energy and protein and even some micronutrients, they may contain too little iron, calcium and other micronutrients, for example iron. Older girls would appear to be at particular risk because of their higher iron needs.

The selection of high fat, sugar-rich snack items as substitutes for more varied meals also poses a threat to long-term health. Children may appear to be healthy because growth is sustained, but the influence of current dietary patterns on health may be more subtle and only evident in the long term.

Some specific problems that may arise in relation to children's eating behaviour are discussed below.

Anaemia

The requirement for iron is high during periods of growth in childhood and particularly in adolescence when large amounts of iron are needed by both sexes for the increases in blood volume, haemoglobin and lean body mass (LBM). The demand for iron in boys is specially high because of the considerable gains in lean body mass and hence adolescent boys are at risk of iron deficiency anaemia (Dallman et al., 1980). Adolescent girls' need for iron increases substantially once menstruation begins and therefore they are at greater risk of iron deficiency than boys (Bailey et al., 1982). The evidence from the dietary studies reviewed earlier reinforces this (see also Part 3, Anaemia in Children and Adults). In girls with substantial blood losses, the Pill can reduce losses by 25%.

Many teenagers are reported to be adopting a vegetarian way of eating and most specifically avoiding red meat, the most readily absorbed source of iron. Although it might be anticipated that such a trend could increase the likelihood of iron deficiency, as yet there is little evidence of its effect on the iron status of teenage girls and young women (see page 76). However, a small study conducted among 12–14 year old girls in London (Nelson et al., 1993) indicated that anaemia was three times more common in vegetarians than omnivores (25% versus 9%), and also in girls who had tried to lose weight in the last year compared with those who had not (23% versus 7%).

The low physical activity levels of many teenagers (see page 52) contribute to low energy intakes, and with this go low intakes of essential nutrients such as iron.

Dental caries

The peak prevalence of dental caries occurs during childhood, with caries occurring in 49% of 5-year-olds and 93% of 15-year-olds (HEA, 1989) (see Chapter 13 and, for a review, Buttriss, 1995).

Obesity

The proportion of overweight and obese adults in Britain has been increasing gradually in recent years. The government's Nutrition Task Force and Physical Activity Task Force are together looking at a means of dealing with this, which is likely to focus on prevention rather than treatment of people who have already become obese. Clearly, a key part of this strategy will be a focus on diet, but a new approach is needed and this will be a concurrent focus on the need to be more physically active.

A number of factors can contribute to overweight and obesity in childhood. These include lack of physical activity, feeding habits in infancy and the preschool years, the influence of emotional factors on eating behaviour and, albeit rarely, hormonal causes and genetic predisposition.

There has been considerable debate as to whether fat children become fat adults. Childhood fatness appears to be a poor predictor of adult obesity when assessed in infancy or before five years of age. However, the risks of adult obesity are greater when overweight is present at age 7–11 years. Braddon and colleagues (1986) showed that 21% of obese 36-year-olds would already have been classified as obese at 11 years, and that weight during the various stages of adolescence was an increasingly good predictor of adult obesity. In addition, overweight or obese young adults usually become much more obese as they age. This means that the risks for future health of overweight young adults are considerably greater than those of overweight middle-aged or elderly people.

The treatment of overweight and obesity in children requires careful handling and has been discussed in detail by Garrow (1988) and Francis (1986). Treatment will depend on the age of the child and the degree of overweight but it is essential that any dietary modification does not prevent normal growth or development of the child. It is also important to avoid isolating the child from the rest of the family; in most cases all can benefit from re-education of family eating patterns. There are obvious dangers in making children, especially girls, unduly conscious of body weight.

The diagnosis of overweight in children is more difficult than in adults. Until the age of 18, centile charts should be used to assess weight for height. The use of standard body mass index (BMI) values is not appropriate for children. Measurements of skinfold thickness are useful in assessing body fatness but are only reliable when carried out by those familiar with the use of the callipers.

In younger children (5–12 years) the aim of treatment should be to prevent overweight progressing to obesity by steering children who have progressed rapidly across weight centile lines back towards the centile compatible with their height. Often it may only be necessary to maintain a steady weight until this becomes appropriate for age, height and sex rather than aiming for actual weight reduction. The principle is to promote energy expenditure by increasing physical activity and to restrict energy intake. Such reductions in energy intake may be achieved by relatively simple manipulations in diet, for example reducing consumption of confectionery, cakes, biscuits, fried foods and fatty foods and including a greater proportion of nutrient-dense foods in the diet. A more severe degree of obesity, where greater dietary restriction is necessary, would require more specialist therapy including the involvement of a qualified dietitian. Garrow (1988) recommends that overweight can best be tackled effectively during the primary school years.

The new approach to the growing problem of overweight and obesity in Britain is prevention rather than cure. Improved liaison between school health services and the primary health care team can help identify children who are overweight or obese, with a view to correcting the imbalance which probably exists in the diet and physical activity patterns of several of the family members, not just the child who has been identified. This approach will help prevent younger children from following a similar path. In general, the 'treatment' is healthy eating advice for the whole family, rather than a special diet for the child. Families in which there is a greater chance of there being an overweight or obese child are often characterized by:

- overweight parents
- single parents
- older parents
- a single child.

Importance of physical activity

Few data exist on the amount of physical activity currently undertaken by children in Britain. Primary schoolchildren seem to remain fairly active in their play (Sleap and Warburton, 1992). However, there is a reduction in physical recreation, particularly in girls, after the age of 12 years (Armstrong et al., 1990).

Fox (1994) concludes that children today seem no less fit, but there is good reason to be concerned about general levels of physical activity, particularly among girls. There is ample evidence that relatively few teenagers engage in the sort of moderate to vigorous activity likely to improve the health of their hearts. Physical activity becomes even more important in adulthood and it is therefore important that teenagers are encouraged to develop interests in a range of pursuits which will still be attractive to them as adults.

An international consensus statement on children's health has concluded that all adolescents should be physically active daily or nearly every day, as part of play, games, sport, work, transportation, or via recreation in the context of the family, school and community. In addition, all adolescents should be involved in three or more sessions per week of activities lasting 20 minutes or more that require moderate to vigorous levels of exertion (Fox, 1994). The rationale for the first set of recommendations is that weight-bearing activity reduces the risk of obesity and enhances bone development, and the rationale for the second recommendation is the associated psychological benefits, and the improvements in blood lipid profile and aerobic fitness. Fox emphasizes the need for health promotion policies that counteract the social pressures which can lead to inactivity.

Perceived overweight

A totally different problem lies in the fact that many people incorrectly perceive themselves to be overweight (see Chapter 12 and Part 3, Eating Disorders). In Balding's (1995) survey of health-related behaviour in young people, 45% of 11–12 year old girls claimed they would like to lose weight and this figure rose to 57% in 15–16 year old girls.

A significant number of boys were also concerned about their body weight being too great: 20%–27%, depending on age. From previous years' surveys they had found that about half of all boys and about three-quarters of girls had made some attempt to lose weight, usually through dieting.

In the DHSS (1989) survey of children's diets, 8% of 14–15 year old girls claimed to be on a diet to lose weight. Results of this study and the study of 15–25 year olds (Bull, 1985) suggest that teenagers on slimming diets are more likely to be short of essential vitamins and minerals than children on higher energy intakes.

In these age groups, self-imposed dieting, particularly when the child is not overweight, is far more likely to precipitate anorexia nervosa than in the adult. If this condition is suspected it will require specialized treatment and the child may have to be referred to a paediatrician and child psychiatrist. Bulimia nervosa is another problem in this age group, the treatment of which again may require referral to specialists in this area. The forces which drive people to seek change in their physical appearance are already evident in children before puberty. Hill and colleagues (1992) have shown that even among nine-year-olds, there are girls who are highly restrained eaters and who report frequent bouts of dieting. On the other hand, adolescent boys are less likely to report dieting, and gaining weight is the wish of one in four boys (Wardle and Marsland, 1990).

It is therefore very important that the promotion of good nutrition among teenagers does not enhance a culture of weight loss, which already leads an unacceptable number of young people to the serious illnesses — anorexia and bulimia nervosa.

The Department of Health and Social Security (1989), Hackett and colleagues (1984), and Woodward (1985) all found that intakes of essential nutrients such as iron and calcium were below the recommended daily amounts in those children whose energy intakes were low. Calcium requirements are high during the teenage years because the amount of calcium in bone almost doubles during the course of adolescence (Matkovic et al., 1990). Low calcium intakes during these important years have been implicated in low bone mass in adulthood and the increased possibility of developing osteoporosis after the menopause.

Vegetarianism

Avoidance of red meat during some stage of childhood is common. This can be due to concern about animal welfare, a dislike of red meat or parental influence. A survey carried out by Gallup on behalf of the Realeat Company (manufacturers of vegetarian foods) found that about 9% of those adults interviewed who had children aged between 6 months and 16 years claimed that their children were vegetarian or avoiding meat (Realeat, 1990). A later survey of over 4000 adults indicated that women were more likely to be non-meat eating than men, particularly in the 16–24 year age group (Realeat, 1993). In this age group, 13% of women claimed to be non-meat eaters (this is three times the national average). Nutritional status will be adequate if care is taken with planning the diet to ensure adequate sources of protein, iron, zinc and B vitamins (see page 75).

Maintaining a good nutritional status on a vegan diet (no foods of animal origin) can be more difficult, particularly for teenagers whose requirements for calcium are very high. It is generally accepted that vegans of all age groups will need vitamin B_{12} supplements (B_{12} is normally obtained from milk and meat). Iron and zinc intakes may also be marginal in teenage vegans but a high vitamin C intake will tend to favour the absorption of these trace minerals.

Vitamins, minerals and IQ

It is well established that frank undernutrition can influence brain function and if sufficiently severe may have permanent effects. In recent years it has been proposed, on the basis of limited evidence, that although a child may not be overtly malnourished, marginal nutritional deficiency might adversely influence mental performance as measured by non-verbal intelligence tests.

In 1988, Benton and Roberts reported a beneficial effect on non-verbal reasoning when vitamin and mineral supplements were given to some pupils. This study attracted criticism of its design, conduct and analysis (Emery et al., 1988) and in 1990 Crombie and colleagues repeated the study with additional features designed to meet the criticisms. The findings of this study did not support those of Benton and Roberts.

A study carried out by Naismith and colleagues also showed no effect of vitamin and mineral supplementation; although younger children were involved in this study, different tests to assess reasoning were used, and a shorter period of and slightly different supplementation were used (Naismith et al., 1988; Nelson et al., 1990).

However, in 1991 the results of a further trial of supplementation conducted in 615 Californian schoolchildren (aged 12–16 years) were published (Schoenthaler et al., 1991a, 1991b). The authors concluded that a multi-vitamin and mineral supplement improved the performance of some children in non-verbal intelligence tests. Once again this paper was the subject of much controversial scientific and public debate and criticism. Most importantly, because data on the diets and nutritional status of the children studied were not published, it is not possible to state whether those who improved on supplementation were in fact deficient in certain nutrients or not.

It remains feasible that a benefit is more likely to be seen in children on poor nutrient intakes (Benton and Buts, 1990). However, it must be concluded at present that whether or not the IQ of a child whose diet is suboptimal in nutrients may be improved by supplementation with selected minerals and vitamins is still unproven. There is a need for further carefully designed studies, which are double-blind and placebo controlled, and which include proper assessment of micro-nutrient intake and status in relation to intellectual performance (Nelson, 1992; Southon et al., 1992). In the meantime, parents should be reassured that if their child is eating adequate amounts of a varied diet which follows the general principles of a healthy diet, and not missing out any key food group, he/she should be deriving the necessary nutrients and not be in need of further supplementation.

Teenage pregnancy

Approximately 1% of all conceptions in England and Wales are in girls under 16 years of age, and of these, 25% are in girls aged 14 years and under (OPCS, 1989). Pregnancy during adolescence imposes additional physiological and emotional stresses. Nutritional requirements will be further increased to meet the additional requirements for the growth and development of the baby. Intake of calcium, iron, zinc, vitamins A and C and folic acid might be inadequate. Nutrient-dense foods such as milk and dairy products, wholegrain cereals, fruit, vegetables, lean meat, poultry, fish and eggs should be emphasized.

Undernutrition

Though relatively rare in the UK, an habitually low food intake will eventually result in undernutrition, which in children manifests as poor growth rates and, in severe cases, as stunting of both physical and perhaps mental development. Although growth failure may occur secondarily to a primary medical condition, undernutrition as a result of poor food intake is rare in the UK. The presence of undernutrition can only be established by the use of anthropometric measures, growth velocity charts and dietary assessment.

Faddy eating in children, specially during adolescence, is common. Although it may be possible to stimulate poor eaters by offering a wider variety of foods, it is generally advisable that the child should not be made aware of concern by parents, friends and medical advisers, as this may simply exacerbate the problem in cases of food avoidance.

The incidence of the eating disorders, anorexia and bulimia nervosa is on the increase. The prevalence is highest in girls from upper socio-economic groups and, in 95% of those affected, appears within five years of puberty (Salmons, 1987). If an eating disorder is suspected, medical advice should be sought (see Part 3, Eating Disorders).

Teenagers: alcohol and tobacco

Large surveys by Balding and colleagues (1988; 1995) have indicated a trend among teenagers of increasing consumption of alcoholic drinks. By the age of 15, the majority of both sexes in the 1994 survey were drinking some alcohol; only 39% of boys and 44% of girls claimed not to have drunk alcohol. The large quantities drunk by some teenagers were particularly worrying — 15% of girls and 26% of boys aged 15–16 years claimed to drink more than 10 units in a week.

The nutritional interactions with alcohol are complex but, as with smoking, alcohol consumption may increase requirements for some nutrients and may adversely influence food intake generally. In addition, alcohol consumption and smoking often go hand in hand.

The high prevalence of regular smoking in young people and the lack of any significant decline in the last decade is alarming (Royal College of Physicians, 1992). A quarter of school leavers (aged 15 years) smoke regularly. It seems that more girls than boys now smoke. This may be associated with perceptions about weight control and maturity. A third of 11-year-olds and two-thirds of 16-year-olds have experimented with smoking. Most adult smokers were regular smokers before the age of 18 years.

Providing a suitable diet

To ensure an adequate supply of nutrients, foods from the four main food groups should be included daily and children should be encouraged to choose a wide variety of foods from these groups. Table 4 (Part 1, page 31) shows the sorts of foods which fall into each of the four groups and provides a suggested number of daily servings, but size of servings will vary depending on appetite, which itself will be influenced by the state of growth in a child.

The general principles of a healthy diet, relatively low in fat, sugar and salt, and relatively high in starch and in non-starch polysaccharide (NSP), as indicated in the COMA report on dietary reference values (DH, 1991), apply to children in this age group. By the time they reach school age, most children should have made the transition to a diet high in starch and non-starch polysaccharide, and lower in fat and simple sugars (see page 37).

A daily pattern of three main meals composed of foods of high nutrient density should be encouraged. The omission of meals may lead to reduced nutrient intakes. Where a child decides to become vegetarian, the risks of anaemia may be high unless the diet is modified in such a way as to include alternative sources of iron (see Part 3, Anaemia in Children and Adults).

Between meals, snacks are often necessary for this age group to meet energy requirements but again these snacks should generally be based on foods of high nutrient density such as bread (preferably wholemeal), toast, sandwiches, breakfast cereal, yogurt, fresh fruit/vegetables, nuts and milk. Items such as confectionery, biscuits, pies, cakes, crisps and soft drinks should not be used as substitutes for more complete meals and should be consumed in moderation.

Eating more healthily may not be a child's highest priority, but motivation can be increased by engaging the child's interest using his or her existing knowledge, for example about sport or appearance. Also, in the family setting, helping in the preparation of food, and using the meal as a learning experience and a social occasion can increase children's interest in improving their diet. The social importance of the eating occasion as a conditioning process for the adoption of appropriate eating habits should not be underestimated.

Booklets on healthy eating written for teenagers are available from the National Dairy Council.

References

Armstrong N et al. (1990) Patterns of physical activity among 11–16 year old British children. *British Medical Journal* **301**, 203–5.

Bailey LB et al. (1982) Serum ferritin as a measure of iron stores in adolescents. *Journal of Pediatrics* **101**, 774–6.

Balding J (1988) *Young People in 1987*. University of Exeter, Health Education Authority/Schools Health Education Unit.

Balding J (1992) *Young People in 1991*. University of Exeter, Schools Health Education Unit.

Balding J (1995) *Young People in 1994*. University of Exeter, Schools Health Education Unit.

Benton D and Roberts G (1988) Effect of vitamin and mineral supplementation on intelligence of sample of schoolchildren. *Lancet* **1**, 140–3.

Benton D and Buts JP (1990) Vitamin/mineral supplementation and intelligence. *Lancet* **335**, 1158–60.

Braddon FEM et al. (1986) Onset of obesity in 36 year birth cohort study. *British Medical Journal* **293**, 299–303.

Bull NL (1985) Dietary habits of 15–25 year olds. *Human Nutrition: Applied Nutrition* **39A**, Suppl. 1, 1–68.

Buttriss J (1995) *Diet and Dental Health*. Topical Update 5. London, National Dairy Council.

Caroline Walker Trust (1992) *Nutritional Guidelines for School Meals*. London, CWT.

Crombie IK et al. (1990) Effect of vitamin and mineral supplementation on verbal and non-verbal reasoning of schoolchildren. *Lancet* **335**, 744–7.

Dallman PR et al. (1980) Iron deficiency in infancy and childhood. *American Journal of Clinical Nutrition* **33**, 86–118.

Department of Health and Social Security, Committee on Medical Aspects of Food Policy (1989) *The Diets of British Schoolchildren. Report on Health and Social Subjects 36*. London, HMSO.

Department of Health, Committee on Medical Aspects of Food Policy (1991) *Dietary Reference Values for Food Energy and Nutrients for the United Kingdom. Report on Health and Social Subjects 41*. London, HMSO.

Emery PW et al. (1988) Vitamin/mineral supplementation and non-verbal intelligence. *Lancet* **1**, 407–9.

Fox KR (1994) Do children take enough exercise? In Buttriss JL (Ed.) *Children in Focus*. Proceedings of a Conference held in 1993. London, National Dairy Council.

Francis DEM (1986) *Nutrition for Children*. Oxford, Blackwell Scientific Publications.

Garrow JS (1988) *Obesity and Related Diseases*. London, Churchill Livingstone.

Hackett AF et al. (1984) A 2 year longitudinal nutritional survey of 405 Northumberland children initially aged 11.5 years. *British Journal of Nutrition* **51**, 67–75.

Health Education Authority (1989) *The Scientific Basis of Dental Health Education*. A policy document. 3rd edn. London, HEA.

Hill AJ et al. (1992) Eating in the adult world: the rise of dieting in childhood and adolescence. *British Journal of Psychology* **23**, 95–105.

Matkovic V et al. (1990) Factors that influence peak bone mass formation: a study of calcium balance and the inheritance of bone mass in adolescent females. *American Journal of Clinical Nutrition* **52**, 878–88.

Naismith DJ et al. (1988) Can children's intelligence be increased by vitamin and mineral supplements? *Lancet* **2**, 335.

Nelson M (1991) Food, vitamins and IQ. *Proceedings of the Nutrition Society* **50**, 29–35.

Nelson M (1992) Vitamin and mineral supplementation and academic performance in school children. *Proceedings of the Nutrition Society* **51**, 303–13.

Nelson M et al. (1990) Nutrient intakes, vitamin-mineral supplementation and intelligence in British schoolchildren. *British Journal of Nutrition* **64**, 13–22.

Nelson M et al. (1993) Haemoglobin, ferritin, and iron intakes in British children aged 12–14 years: a preliminary investigation. *British Journal of Nutrition* **70**, 147–55.

Office of Population Censuses and Surveys (1989) *Birth Statistics 1987*. London, HMSO.

Realeat (1990) *Changing Attitudes to Meat Consumption*. London, Realeat.

Realeat (1993) *Changing Attitudes to Meat Consumption*. London, Realeat.

Royal College of Physicians (1992) *Smoking and the Young*. London, RCP.

Rugg-Gunn AJ et al. (1991) Empty calories? Nutrient intake in relation to sugar intake in English adolescents. *Journal of Human Nutrition and Dietetics* **4**, 101–11.

Salmons PH (1987) Anorexia nervosa and related conditions in schoolchildren. *Nutrition and Health* **4**, 217–25.

Schoenthaler SJ et al. (1991a) Controlled trial of vitamin-mineral supplementation on intelligence and brain function. *Personality and Individual Differences* **12**, 343–50.

Schoenthaler SJ et al. (1991b) Controlled trial of vitamin-mineral supplementation: effects on intelligence and performance. *Personality and Individual Differences* **12,** 351–62.

Sleap M and Warburton P (1992) Physical activity levels in 5–11 year old children in England as determined by continuous observation. *Research Quarterly for Exercise and Sport* **63,** 238–45.

Southon S et al. (1992) Micronutrient intake and psychological performance of schoolchildren: consideration of the value of calculated nutrient intakes for the assessment of micronutrient status in children. *Proceedings of the Nutrition Society* **51,** 315–24.

Wardle J and Marsland L (1990) Adolescent concerns about weight and eating: a social-developmental perspective. *Journal of Psycho-somatic Research* **34,** 377–91.

Woodward DR (1985) What sort of teenager has low intakes of energy and nutrients? *British Journal of Nutrition* **51,** 67–75.

Further reading

Buttriss J and Gray J (1995) *Nutrition and Teenagers. Fact File 5 (Revised).* London, NDC.

5

Elderly people

Key points

1. The maintenance of good nutrition contributes to health and well-being and recovery from trauma and illness among elderly people.

2. Energy requirements decline in old age, because of loss of lean tissue and consequent reduction in basal metabolic rate, and because elderly people are less active. But if energy intake is maintained the diet is more likely to provide adequate nutrients. Therefore, moderate physical activity should be vigorously promoted as a means of maintaining muscle mass and hence energy requirements. There is need for a change in emphasis with regard to exercise.

3. The diets of elderly people should contain a wide variety of foods of high nutrient density (high ratio of nutrients to calories). As with younger adults, the majority of people over 65 should aim to eat more foods rich in starch and non-starch polysaccharides (dietary fibre) and less fat and simple sugars. But these guidelines may not be appropriate for the very elderly or for the chronically sick, for whom quantity and energy density, as well as quality, of food will be very important.

4. The nutritional status of elderly people may be influenced by a range of factors including socio-economic ones and there is risk of malnutrition in some elderly people. More attention should be given to the nutritional intake and status of elderly people in long-stay care in hospitals and nursing homes.

5. Both osteoporosis and osteomalacia are more common in elderly people. Although increases in the intake of calcium cannot restore lost bone in osteo-porosis, it is important to maintain an adequate intake of the mineral. Maintenance of physical activity levels is also essential. In order to maintain adequate levels of vitamin D, exposure to summer sunlight and consumption of foods rich in vitamin D should be encouraged. Those who are housebound or institutionalized will require supplementation to bring their daily intake up to 10 µg per day.

6. Interactions between drug therapy and nutrition are more likely to occur in elderly people.

7. There is a need to be aware of the adverse risks of both overweight and underweight in elderly people.

8. Fluid intake, equivalent to at least eight cups per day, is important to avoid dehydration and associated problems.

In contrast to other population groups, elderly people are a particularly heterogeneous group because of physiological, medical and social diversity. Actual chronological age may not reflect the state of health and therefore the nutritional needs of the individual. Many factors can influence the nutritional status of older people and nutritional factors are often secondary to social, emotional, economic or cultural factors as well as illness and disability. There needs to be greater awareness that maintaining good nutrition in elderly people can make an important contribution to both health and well-being and recovery from illness in this group.

Nutritional needs

With the exception of vitamin D, there are no specific dietary reference values (DRVs) for elderly people, since nutritional needs are generally thought to be similar to those of younger adults (aged over 50 years) (see Part 1, Appendix 2). However, energy requirements are generally reduced as a result of lower levels of physical activity and a decrease in metabolic rate as lean tissue is lost. To avoid obesity, past eating habits may need to be adjusted to accommodate these changes, but as nutrient requirements are the same, or may even be increased, more attention has to be given to dietary quality or nutrient density (the quantity of nutrients in relation to calories).

The COMA Working Group on the Nutrition of Elderly People recommended that similar patterns of eating and lifestyle to those advised for younger adults for the maintenance of health should be adopted by the majority of people aged 65 years or more (DH, 1992). The importance of the maintenance of physical activity for muscle tone and power should not be under-estimated (see page 61). Higher levels of physical activity result in higher energy expenditure, which in turn permits a higher energy intake and therefore a higher food intake, thereby making it easier to obtain necessary nutrients.

In terms of food components, the working group recommended that elderly people should reduce intakes of fat and simple sugars whilst increasing their intakes of starchy foods, non-starch polysaccharides (fibre) and vitamin D. The need for diets which provide a variety of nutrient-dense foods was emphasized.

In general, elderly people should be encouraged to adopt diets aimed to reduce plasma cholesterol level on the basis of an association between plasma cholesterol and risk of coronary heart disease. Contrary to earlier data from the Framingham study (Gofman et al., 1966), recent data suggest that although the relative risk of coronary heart disease associated with plasma cholesterol declines with age, the level of blood cholesterol remains a predictor up to and possibly beyond the age of 70 years (Gordon and Rifkind, 1989).

However, in practical terms it should be emphasized that although these recommendations should be promoted for younger elderly people, it is not realistic or even appropriate to attempt to make drastic changes in the relative fat content of the diets of those aged 85 and above, provided they are not obese, or in those who are chronically sick. However, it would appear to be beneficial to encourage **all** elderly people to consume regularly oily fish such as mackerel, sardines, salmon, and pilchards, as a source of n-3 fatty acids, in order to reduce the risk of thrombosis (DH, 1992).

Use of diuretics is common among elderly people. This can cause potassium depletion, which in turn can result in weakness and mental confusion (see pages 64 and 66). It is therefore important that potassium-rich foods such as fruit (especially bananas), fruit juice, potatoes and vegetables are eaten regularly (see Part 1, Appendix 2 for a more complete list).

Malnutrition in elderly people

Nutrition surveys of non-institutionalized elderly people in Britain (DHSS, 1972, 1979) have shown that elderly people who are in good health typically have similar dietary patterns and eat similar foods to younger people. However, more up-to-date information on the diets and nutritional status of elderly people is needed. Such information will become available in due course from a study planned as part of the National Diet and Nutrition Survey programme (a joint venture of MAFF and DH). Fieldwork for this study began in 1994.

In the initial DHSS survey carried out in 1967/68, 3% of those surveyed were shown to be suffering from malnutrition, which in three-quarters of the cases was associated with clinical disease (DHSS, 1972). In a second survey of the surviving participants of the earlier study, carried out in 1972/73 (DHSS, 1979), 7% of these elderly people were diagnosed as being malnourished. The prevalence of malnutrition was greater in those over 80 years of age. Most of these people were suffering from an energy deficit

Table 5.1 *Factors contributing to malnutrition in elderly people*

Primary	Secondary
★ Ignorance (about food and nutrition)	★ Impaired appetite
★ Poverty	★ Poor dentition
★ Mental disturbance	★ Reduced absorption
★ Physical disability	★ Alcohol abuse
★ Chronic disease states, e.g. bronchitis	★ Smoking
★ Social isolation and loneliness, leading to apathy and depression	★ Drug therapy

Source: Adapted from Exton-Smith (1971).

but deficiencies of vitamin B$_{12}$, folic acid, iron and even cases of frank scurvy were observed.

There is evidence from a study in Southampton that housebound elderly people may be at greater risk of deficiencies of protein, calcium, phosphorus, iron, zinc, copper and selenium compared to healthy and free-living elderly people (Thomas et al., 1988; Bunker and Clayton, 1989). Studies of elderly people in both hospital and residential homes indicate that food intakes are generally less than those reported in free-living elderly people (DH, 1992). The Southampton studies have shown that the long-stay geriatric patients studied generally had low energy intakes and consistently lost weight over a one-year period (Thomas et al., 1988).

Although clinical signs of frank malnutrition are rare in elderly people, the influence of marginal or sub-nutrition on the health and well-being of the elderly could be considerable. Fractured bones, leg ulcers, pressure sores and an increased susceptibility to infection are common problems in elderly people. The role of vitamins, minerals and especially trace minerals, such as zinc and copper, in the healing process and in resistance to infection is likely to be important (Thomas et al., 1988).

The COMA Working Group emphasized the need to assess routinely elderly people admitted to hospital and to provide supplements to improve nutritional status during their hospital stay, especially following trauma or surgery (DH, 1992). The working group also highlighted the need for awareness of inadequate food intake of elderly people in institutions and the need for proper investigation of the impact of acute and chronic illness on the nutritional requirements of elderly people.

Various risk factors which contribute to malnutrition in elderly people have been identified. These were divided into primary and secondary risk factors more than twenty years ago by Exton-Smith (1971) — a classification which is still relevant (Table 5.1). When several of these factors operate in concert, there is a high risk of malnutrition developing.

A list of seven markers of potential poor nutrition have been identified (adapted from Davies, 1984):

- Eating fewer than eight main meals a week (a 'main' meal should include foods from at least three of the four main food groups; see Appendix 1 and Part 1, page 31)

- Drinking less than half a pint of milk per day (or alternatives: a yogurt or 1$\frac{1}{2}$ oz hard cheese is equivalent, in terms of calcium, to one-third of a pint of milk)

- Absence in the diet or infrequent consumption of fruit and vegetables (see Part 1, page 32)

- Leaving or wasting food, including meals on wheels

- Long periods in the day (more than five hours) without food and drink

- Depressed or lonely

- Unexpected weight change (gain or loss).

Risk factors and warning signals such as these have been incorporated into a check-list (Table 5.2) which can be used to assess elderly clients both in the community and on entry to residential homes and institutional care (Davies and Knutson, 1991). The grid system allows risk factors found in a particular client or patient to be evaluated in the light of observed warning signals. For example, someone who is living alone is likely to become malnourished if one or more of the warning signals in the 'living alone' column is present.

After observing the interaction of risk factors and warning signals, the next step is practical action, as illustrated in Figure 5.1. Further examples of methods of preventive care among elderly people can be found in a review by Taylor and Buckley (1988).

Need for more physical activity

The Department of Health recommendations (1992) have placed particular emphasis on the need for elderly people to be more active, in order to:

- improve muscle tone and power
- improve well-being (psychological health)
- improve cardiovascular fitness
- keep joints mobile
- enable greater energy (and thereby nutrient) consumption
- improve recovery from illness.

Current perceptions of the value of physical activity for older people need to be changed.

Table 5.2 *Relevant risk factors and observed warning signals*

Warning signals	Living alone	House-bound	No regular cooked meals	Low mental test score	Clinical diagnosis of depression	Chronic bronchitis/ emphysema	Gastrectomy	Poor definition and/or difficulty in swallowing
Risk factors								
Recent unintended weight change ± 3 kg (7 lb)	•	•	•	•	•	•	•	•
Physical disability affecting food shopping, preparation, or intake	•	•	•		•	•		
Lack of sunlight		•			•			
Bereavement and/or observed depression/loneliness	•	•		•	•	•		
Mental confusion affecting eating	•		•	•				
High alcohol consumption	•		•		•			
Multiple medications/long-term medication	•			•	•			
Missed meals, snacks, fluids	•	•	•	•	•	•	•	•
Food wastage/rejection	•	•	•	•	•	•		•
Insufficient food stores at home	•	•	•	•	•	•		
Lack of fruits, juices, vegetables in diet	•	•	•					•
Low budget for food	•		•					
Poor nutritional knowledge		•	•	•			•	•

Source: Davies L and Knutson CK (1991). Warning signals for malnutrition in the elderly. © American Dietetic Association. Reprinted by permission of the *Journal of the American Dietetic Association* **91,** 1413–7.

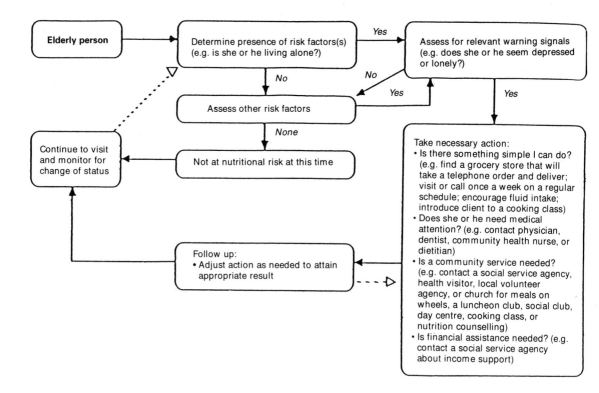

Figure 5.1 *Application of warning signal concept*
Source: Davies L and Knutson CK (1991). Warning signals for malnutrition in the elderly. © American Dietetic Association. Reprinted by permission of the *Journal of the American Dietetic Association* **91**, 1413–7.

A physically active life is beneficial and, barring serious illness, possible well into the eighth decade of life.

Prompt resumption of activity after episodes of intercurrent illness should be encouraged. Inactivity associated with minor illness often leads to loss of muscle tone and mass, and this can result in a stepwise decline in physical fitness, which is sometimes assumed by individuals and their families to be inevitable.

Many elderly people spend no more than an hour per day on their feet (DH, 1992) and so encouraging them to be on their feet more is a good start. Other suitable activities include: gardening, walking, dancing, gentle keep fit, cycling, swimming, housework and house maintenance. As with all age groups, the increase in physical activity should be gradual and appropriate to ability.

Role of nutrition in common problems

Drug-nutrient interactions

Most of the chronic diseases which prevail in the elderly, for example hypertension and arthritis, require continual medication, so the use of prescribed drugs is especially high in this group. Non-prescription drugs, including analgesics, antacids and laxatives, are also used widely by this group. It is therefore likely that a range of drug-drug and drug-nutrient interactions may occur in the elderly (Roe, 1988), particularly as polypharmacy is a fact of life for many elderly people.

It is well recognized that the ageing process itself may influence drug metabolism, for example because of changes in gastro-intestinal, hepatic and renal function. It may

Table 5.3 *Mechanisms responsible for drug effects on nutrient absorption with examples of each*

	Drug	Change in nutrient absorption
Primary effect		
Intraluminal interaction		
Absorption	Cholestyramine	↓ folate
Precipitation	Aluminium hydroxide	↓ phosphate
Chelation	Tetracycline	↓ calcium
Solubilization	Mineral oil	↓ beta-carotene
Change in pH	Sodium bicarbonate	↓ folate
Enzyme inhibition	Sulfasalazine	↓ folate
Change in motility		
Slowed gastric emptying	Anticholinergic drugs	↑ riboflavin
Shortened intestinal transit	Acarbose	↓ sugars
Mucosal damage		
Cytotoxicity	Neomycin	
	Colchicine	↓ fat
	Methotrexate	↓ calcium
Secondary effect		
Due to maldigestion	Alcohol — impaired bile acid secretion	↓ fat
Due to non-gastro-intestinal enzyme inhibition	Isoniazid — reduces hepatic hydroxylation of vitamin D to active metabolite	↓ calcium due to inhibition of vitamin D metabolism
Due to drug-induced vitamin deficiency	Alcohol — folate deficiency leads to abnormal enterocytes	↓ thiamin due to folate metabolism

Source: Adapted from Roe (1985).

be less well recognized, however, that the reduced lean body mass in most elderly people means that drug doses may need to be reduced. Coupled with polypharmacy and subclinical disease, the drugs elderly people take may actually be making them feel ill.

It is also known that certain drugs can influence nutritional status and consequently may alter the requirement for a particular nutrient. Some drugs influence sense of taste, appetite and therefore food and nutrient intake. These effects compound the reduction in the senses of taste and smell which often occur with ageing (Schiffman, 1993). They may also cause a rise in consumption of flavouring agents such as salt and sugar, both of which could have adverse effects on health.

Many drugs, including alcohol, influence the absorption, metabolism and elimination of nutrients. Drinking alcohol seems to slow down metabolism of drugs taken concurrently, presumably because of competition for substrate binding sites in the liver. However, in the chronic drinker, with chronically elevated concentrations of enzymes to metabolize ethanol, abstention from alcohol on the day a drug is taken can accelerate normal metabolism of the drug (Lieber, 1988). Clearly these effects could interfere with the body's handling of drugs and hence be

Table 5.4 *Drugs which may affect mineral and vitamin metabolism*

Drug	Possible effect
Anticonvulsants	Interference with vitamin D metabolism and folate absorption
Biguanides	Reduce vitamin B_{12} and folate status
Prolonged aspirin usage	Tissue depletion of ascorbic acid; can induce bleeding in the gastro-intestinal tract, resulting in iron deficiency anaemia
Thiazide diuretics	Can result in potassium depletion and magnesium and zinc deficiency
Anti-cancer drug	Can reduce thiamin status

associated with a variety of side-effects, including enhanced or reduced effectiveness of the drug.

Absorption effects may occur as a direct consequence of changes in intraluminal or mucosal factors, or motility, or be secondary to, for example, the effect of the drug on hepatic metabolism of nutrients (Table 5.3). Table 5.4 lists further adverse effects of some drugs on nutrient metabolism.

There is extensive information derived from animal studies and some more limited information from human studies, which indicates that drug metabolism can be influenced by various nutritional factors, including protein and ascorbic acid. However, few studies of these interrelationships have been undertaken in elderly people (Anderson, 1990).

Immune function

In some elderly people, immune function will be compromised by the drugs they are taking, for example long-term steroids, or by subclinical disease. Work in Canada has indicated that illness due to infections was cut by half in those elderly people whose intake of nutrients

was in line with dietary recommendations (Chandra, 1992).

Cataracts

There is growing interest in the potential of antioxidant nutrients, such as vitamin E and beta-carotene, to reduce the incidence and progress of cataracts among elderly people (Packer, 1991). This underlines the importance of a nutrient-rich diet and, in particular, a good intake of fruit and vegetables (see Appendix 1 and Part 1, page 31).

Constipation

Constipation is a common problem in the elderly, believed to occur in about 20% of people aged 65 years and over (DH, 1991). Inactivity coupled with a low food intake and use of laxatives can exacerbate the problem. The most appropriate treatment for non-drug induced constipation is dietary modification coupled with moderate regular exercise, which is usually more effective than lactulose, for example.

Some elderly people have very low intakes of non-starch polysaccharides (NSP) associated with their low energy intakes. There is good evidence that increased intake can prevent and relieve constipation and an average 50% increase in NSP intake was recommended (DH, 1991). The COMA Working Group advise that comparable intakes are appropriate for most elderly people (DH, 1992). However it cautions against the excessive use of foods with a high phytate content, especially raw bran, as this reduces the absorption of calcium, iron, copper and zinc.

A gradual increase in NSP intake over a period of a couple of weeks, from a range of sources but particularly wholegrain cereals, vegetables and fruit, should be encouraged (see Part 1, page 33 for ways to increase NSP intake). An increase in fluid intake should also be recommended, both to promote bowel action and to reduce the risk of obstruction. Raw bran is no longer recommended. Also, by taking more exercise, more food can be consumed without increasing body weight, and this will automatically increase faecal bulk.

Bone health

Osteoporosis is prevalent in middle and old age, especially in women, and it is becoming more common. It has been estimated to affect one in four women over the age of 60 years and one in two over 75 years. Its association with increased fracture rates, especially of the femoral neck, has high morbidity, mortality and economic costs.

The precise role of dietary calcium in the pathogenesis of osteoporosis is still unclear. Although there is increasing evidence that low dietary calcium intakes in childhood and young adulthood may be associated with a reduced peak bone mass (Kanders et al., 1988; Matkovic et al., 1990), the influence of calcium intake on bone mass in elderly people is uncertain.

However, it is important, as stressed by the COMA Working Group to ensure that dietary calcium intakes should not fall below current levels (DH, 1992). Milk and milk products are important sources of dietary calcium and households of elderly people do usually consume more milk than other households. The contribution of dairy products to calcium intake is discussed in Part 1 (page 46). The importance of sustaining adequate levels of physical activity in maintaining the bone health of elderly people must be stressed.

A variety of other lifestyle factors have been linked with increased risk of osteoporosis, including smoking, high salt intake, and high alcohol intake (Smith, 1990). For further information see Chapter 11.

Osteomalacia due to impaired mineralization of the skeleton is the clinical manifestation of vitamin D deficiency in adults. It may also lead to increased fracture rates in the elderly, but there are limited data on its prevalence (DH, 1992).

Vitamin D status may be low in the elderly for a number of reasons. It may be reduced because of malabsorption or gastric surgery or as a result of abnormal hepatic metabolism because of anticonvulsant therapy or liver disease. However, because the major source of vitamin D is via skin synthesis, elderly people with reduced mobility or who are housebound or institutionalized may be unable to achieve the necessary levels of synthesis.

It has been demonstrated that limited exposure (hands, forearms and face) to even short periods of summer sunlight (15–30 minutes per day) can supply adequate amounts of vitamin D (Holick, 1990) and this should be recommended for all elderly people. However, good dietary sources of the vitamin should also be encouraged for all elderly people (see Part 1, page 45).

Average intakes of vitamin D from diet are about 2.0 µg/day. Provision of vitamin D supplements is recommended for elderly people who are housebound or institutionalized, in a dose which provides a total daily intake of 10 µg (DH, 1992). This may be given as a daily supplement or as six-monthly or annual depot injections.

Overweight and obesity

Almost half of the adult British population is overweight (OPCS, 1993) but body mass index (BMI), defined as weight in kilograms divided by height squared in metres, peaks at about age 65, on average. Table 5.5 shows the prevalence of underweight (BMI under 20), overweight (BMI over 25) and obesity (BMI over 30) in men and women over age 65. It should be noted that the assumption that the BMI ranges used for younger adults are also appropriate for elderly people, who usually have less lean mass, has been questioned (for example, Andres et al., 1985). However, an alternative system for assessment is yet to be validated.

Being overweight or obese will exacerbate existing cardio-respiratory problems, and put extra strain on and worsen pain in arthritic joints, particularly knees, in elderly people. It may also precipitate non-insulin dependent diabetes (regardless of BMI, the chances of adult-onset diabetes developing can be reduced by taking regular exercise). Moreover, excess weight is likely to restrict activity levels leading to a reduction in muscle mass, which will itself lead to further reduction in

Table 5.5 *Prevalence of underweight, overweight and obesity among elderly people*

Age (years)	Underweight (BMI < 20) %	Overweight (BMI > 25) %	Obese (BMI > 30) %
Men: 65–74	3	45	14
Men: 75+	8	46	7
Women: 65–74	6	41	19
Women: 75+	7	36	16

Source: OPCS (1993).

basal metabolic rate and thus in energy requirement.

Advice to maintain physical activity levels (gardening, housework, walking), together with specific advice on diet, may be necessary to help elderly people to control their weight (see page 62). However, dietary advice must be designed to ensure that any reduction in dietary energy does not lead to a concomitant reduction in nutrient density of the diet.

Underweight

The COMA Working Group drew attention to the problem of underweight (DH, 1992). Elderly people who are underweight are particularly susceptible to intercurrent illness and trauma, because of a lack of metabolic reserves to deal with the additional stress. Excess morbidity and mortality are associated with low body mass in old age (Campbell et al., 1990).

Slow progressive weight loss may be overlooked and it is important to be aware that thin elderly people are likely to have been consuming a diet that is not only energy deficient, but inadequate in nutrients too.

Dehydration

Dehydration may occur in the elderly because of the recognized diminution in the thirst response and because older people may cut down on fluids to avoid frequent urination or because of fear of incontinence. Diuretic therapy can compound the situation and may also lead to hypokalaemia (low blood potassium). The resultant symptoms of mental confusion, headaches, irritability and weak-

ness may go unnoticed (see page 59). Fluid intake should be the equivalent of at least eight cups per day.

Improving nutritional status

There is a need for studies to determine both the micronutrient intake and biochemical status of elderly people and the contribution of a deficiency of certain micronutrients to physical and psychological problems in this population group (DH, 1992). There is increasing evidence that the antioxidant nutrients (vitamins C, E, A, beta-carotene, selenium, zinc and copper) may protect against various degenerative disorders (see page 64) and therefore elderly people, like the rest of the population, should be encouraged to eat more vegetables, fruit and wholegrain cereals as sources of these nutrients, as well as of non-starch polysaccharides. Particular attention should be given to ensuring adequate vitamin C consumption, especially in those who are institutionalized (DH, 1992).

Practical advice

Developing and maintaining an interest in food is essential if nutritional status is to be sustained or improved, as this will result in a more varied and balanced diet. This can be achieved by:
- eating with friends and sharing the cooking for those living alone, or attending luncheon clubs
- adapting cookery and utensils if problems such as arthritis make preparing and eating food difficult
- replacing ill-fitting dentures

- adjusting to a pattern of small but more frequent meals to suit the reduced appetites of some elderly people.

Food packed in small quantities tends to be more expensive and those living alone may have particular financial difficulties. Convenience foods may be a new concept for some elderly people and advice on their use may be needed. However, there are many economical and nutritious dishes that can be produced using a few basic nutrient-rich foods such as bread and other cereals, vegetables and fruit, milk and its products, and fish and meat. Advice on appropriate store cupboard/freezer foods to maintain a healthy diet is helpful.

References

Anderson KE (1990) Nutritional effects on hepatic drug metabolism in the elderly. In Prinsley DM and Stanstead HH (Eds) *Nutrition and Ageing. Progress in Clinical and Biological Research* **326**, 263–77.

Andres R et al. (1985) Impact of age on weight goals. *Annals of Internal Medicine* **103**, 1030–3.

Bunker VW and Clayton BE (1989) Studies on the nutrition of elderly people with particular reference to essential trace elements. *Age and Ageing* **18**, 422–9.

Campbell AJ et al. (1990) Anthropometic measurements as predictors of mortality in a community population aged 70 years and over. *Age and Ageing* **19**, 131–5.

Chandra RK (1992) Effect of vitamin and trace element supplements on immune responses and infection in early subjects. *Lancet* **340**, 1124–7.

Davies L (1984) Nutrition and the elderly: identifying those at risk. *Proceedings of the Nutrition Society* **43**, 295–332.

Davies L and Knutson CK (1991) Warning signals for malnutrition in the elderly. *Journal of the American Dietetic Association* **91**, 1413–7.

Department of Health (1991) *Dietary Reference Values for Food Energy and Nutrients for the UK. Report on Health and Social Subjects 43.* London, HMSO.

Department of Health, Committee on Medical Aspects of Food Policy (1992) *The Nutrition of Elderly People. Report on Health and Social Subjects 43.* London, HMSO.

Department of Health and Social Security (1972) *A Nutrition Survey of the Elderly. Reports on Health and Social Subjects 3.* London, HMSO.

Department of Health and Social Security (1979) *Nutrition and Health in Old Age. Report on Health and Social Subjects 16.* London, HMSO.

Exton-Smith AN (1971) Nutrition of the elderly. *British Journal of Hospital Medicine* **5**, 639–46.

Gofman JW et al. (1966) Ischemic heart disease, atherosclerosis and longevity. *Circulation* **34**, 679–97.

Gordon DJ and Rifkind BM (1989) Treating high blood cholesterol in the older patient. *American Journal of Cardiology* **63**, 48H–52H.

Holick MF (1990) The intimate relationship between the sun, skin and vitamin D: a new perspective. *Bone: Clinical and Biochemical News and Reviews* **7**, 66–69.

Kanders B et al. (1988) Interaction of calcium nutrition and physical activity on bone mass in young people. *Journal of Bone Mineral Research* **3**, 145–9.

Lieber CS (1988) Biochemical and molecular basis of alcohol-induced injury to liver and other tissues. *New England Journal of Medicine* **319**, 1639–50.

Matkovic V et al. (1990) Factors that influence peak bone mass formation; a study of calcium balance and the inheritance of bone mass in adolescent females. *American Journal of Clinical Nutrition* **52**, 878–88.

Office of Population Censuses and Surveys (1993) *Health Survey for England 1991.* A survey carried out by the Social Survey Division of OPCS on behalf of the Department of Health. London, HMSO.

Packer L (1991) Protective role of vitamin E in biological systems. *American Journal of Clinical Nutrition* **53**, 1050S–1055S.

Roe DA (1985) Drug effects on nutrient absorption, transport, and metabolism. *Drug-Nutrient Interactions* **4**, 117–35.

Roe DA (1988) Diet, nutrition and drug reactions. In Shils ME et al. (Eds) *Modern Nutrition in Health and Disease.* Philadelphia, Lea and Febiger. pp 630–45.

Schiffman SS (1993) Food acceptability and nutritional status: considerations for the ageing population in the 21st century. In Leathwood P et al. (Eds) *For a Better Nutrition in the 21st Century.* Nestlé Nutrition Workshop Series, Vol. 27. New York, Nestec Vevey/Raven Press.

Smith R (1990) *Osteoporosis 1990.* London, Royal College of Physicians.

Taylor RC and Buckley EG (Eds) (1988) *Preventive Care of the Elderly: A Review of Current Developments. Occasional Paper 35.* London, Royal College of General Practitioners.

Thomas AJ et al. (1988) Energy, protein, zinc and copper status of twenty one elderly in-patients: analysed dietary intake, metabolic balance studies and biochemical status. *British Journal of Nutrition* **59**, 181–91.

Further reading

Buttriss JL and Gray J (1992) *Nutrition and Elderly People. Fact File 9.* London, National Dairy Council.

Section 2:
Social Aspects of Nutrition

6

Religious restrictions and cultural beliefs

Key points

1. Whatever the ethnic or cultural background in which it is eaten, food not only plays a role in maintaining good health but it may also have a very important social and religious significance.

2. Most of the diets chosen for religious reasons are likely to be nutritionally adequate provided that sufficient food is eaten.

3. Where dietary change is required, advice should be tailored to the person's customary eating pattern.

4. Whilst it is possible to give guidelines on the food habits of different groups, it must be remembered that these are not representative of every member of a particular ethnic group. Only a brief outline is given here.

Food rules and fasting patterns

Food preferences often depend on the area from which a particular community originates, but the religious group determines which foods are forbidden and when and how they should fast (Table 6.1).

In Britain, food restrictions are often completely retained by those who are very religious, and any suggestion that they should consume foods not eaten for religious reasons may cause offence. However, food rules are often relaxed by individuals who have adopted more 'Westernized' eating habits. The food patterns of ethnic minority groups may be affected in a variety of ways:

- Traditional foods may not be available
- Traditional foods may be expensive
- Women may work and therefore not have the time to prepare traditional dishes.

In health terms, the Westernization of traditional diets may be disadvantageous. For example, regular consumption of a variety of fresh fruit and vegetables is generally a part of the diet of many people from ethnic minority communities. However, this may not always be maintained in Britain owing to the expense of imported foods. Although the older generation may maintain traditional eating patterns, it appears that the diets of the younger generation are changing to include more sugar, fat and processed foods, such as fizzy drinks, pies, biscuits, crisps and takeaways.

Information on healthy eating in the context of traditional dietary patterns can be found on pages 88–89.

Food belief systems

Some people of non-Western cultures follow food practices based on traditional ideas about health. These may depend on food availability, the person's physiological state, or concepts of health and disease; they are often influenced by religious restrictions (see page 72). Two such practices include the 'hot' and 'cold' concept and the 'Yin' and 'Yang' concept.

'Hot' and 'cold' concept

The concept of 'hot' and 'cold' food is followed by many people from Bangladesh,

Table 6.1 *Outline of the food rules and fasting patterns in eight religions according to strict interpretation of religious beliefs*

Religion	Foods which may be avoided	Fasting rules
Muslim	Pork, non-halal meat and chicken Shellfish* Alcohol **Meat from animals and birds must be killed according to Muslim law (halal)**	Required to fast from dawn to sunset during the month of Ramadan, the ninth month of the Muslim calendar **Exemptions:** elderly people and children under 12; women who are pregnant, breast feeding or menstruating, and people who are ill or travelling are temporarily exempt and must fast at an alternative time
Hindu	Meat (some eat lamb, chicken) Fish (some eat white fish) Eggs Alcohol	Some devout Hindus will fast[†] for one or two days a week from dawn to sunset; some will take fluids only and others will eat fruit and yogurt which are considered to be pure
Sikh	Beef, pork Some are vegetarian Alcohol	Some devout Sikhs fast[†] once or twice a week
Buddhist	Chicken, lamb, pork, beef Shellfish* (some avoid all fish) Alcohol	No specific belief about fasting
Rastafarian	Pork Shellfish Some are vegetarian Alcohol, coffee, tea	No specific belief about fasting
Jewish	Pork Shellfish* **Animals and birds must be slaughtered by the Jewish method. The meat is then salted and soaked to remove blood and render it kosher (permitted). Meat and milk or milk products must not be served at the same meal or cooked together**	Yom Kippur is a fast day in September or October Passover is celebrated over eight days in April and commemorates the Exodus of Jews from Egypt. At this time leavened bread may be avoided; unleavened bread (matzos) and cakes and biscuits from matzo meal are eaten instead
Seventh day adventist	Pork Shellfish* Alcohol, coffee, tea, cocoa Most avoid eggs and milk and milk products, and some are vegetarian	No specific beliefs about fasting
Mormon	Alcohol, coffee, tea	No specific belief about fasting

*All fish without fins and scales
[†]The strictness of the fast depends on individual preference, and only specific foods may be avoided. The definition of fasting should be further investigated with each person to determine the degree of restriction.

Table 6.2 *Typical 'hot' and 'cold' foods*

'Hot' foods		'Cold' foods
These are pungent, acidic or salty		**These are sweet, bitter, sour or astringent**
Meat	Aubergine	Cereals including rice, bread, chapatti
Fish	Dates	Potato
Lentils	Mango	Milk and milk products
Eggs	Papaya	Fruit
Carrots	Some spices★	Leafy vegetables
Onions	Honey	Nuts
Capsicum	Tea	Some spices★

★'Hot' spices: chilli powder, cinnamon, cloves, garlic, ginger, mustard, nutmeg, pepper.
 'Cold' spices: coriander, cumin, cardomon, fennel, tamarind.

India and Pakistan and may have strong influences on a person's choice of food.

Classification is based on the effect that food has on the body, and its taste. In general, the temperature or spiciness of the food is not considered. Some people believe that certain foods raise the body temperature and excite emotions whereas others lower the body temperature and calm the emotions. Sometimes, illness, diseases and physiological states are defined as 'hot' or 'cold' conditions, and eating the appropriate foods helps to restore the balance. For example, in some communities, pregnancy is regarded as a 'hot condition' and eating predominantly 'cold' foods restores the balance in the body (see Chapter 1 for nutritional requirements). Another belief is that with a healthy person, eating 'hot' and 'cold' foods in excess or at the wrong time can have a bad effect.

Typical 'hot' and 'cold' foods are given in Table 6.2. However, foods that are considered 'hot' by some people may be considered 'cold' by others. Provided that a variety of foods are consumed, this style of eating should not lead to nutritional deficiencies.

Yin and yang concept

In traditional Chinese medicine, good health depends on maintaining a balance in the body of two opposite elements: 'yin' (cold) and 'yang' (hot). When someone's 'equilibrium' is altered, he or she becomes ill and the body becomes too hot (an excess of yang) or too cold (an excess of yin). Diet plays an important role in helping people to maintain a normal healthy balance (Table 6.3).

Table 6.3 *A general guide to foods that have 'heating' (yang) and 'cooling' (yin) properties*★

Hot foods (Yang)	Neutral foods (Yin Yang)	Cold foods (Yin)
Red meat	White fish, e.g. haddock, cod	Chicken
Oily fish, e.g. mackerel, salmon	Rice	Fruit
Herbs	Some vegetables	Some vegetables, e.g. green vegetables
Spices	Steamed food	Boiled or stir-fried food
Alcoholic drinks		
Oils and fats		
Roast and deep-fried food		

★The main food in a dish is also affected by the other foods it is cooked with.

Macrobiotic diets

Macrobiotics originated in Japan early this century and is based on the 'yin yang' theory. The philosophy behind this regimen stems from a number of Eastern religions, but particularly Zen Buddhism. In its most extreme form, the diet is very restricted, consisting of cereal (brown rice) only.

In general, the diet consists of whole grain cereals such as brown rice, whole wheat, maize, barley and buckwheat. Beans, soya products, fresh and preferably organic vegetables and seaweeds can be added. Some fish, poultry, eggs and fruit may be eaten occasionally. Fluids are also restricted.

Nutritional deficiencies can develop, and infants and young children are particularly at risk (Sams, 1972; Francis, 1986). Miller and colleagues (1991) studied the vitamin B_{12} status of a macrobiotic community in New England. Fifty-five per cent of the children studied had indications of low tissue vitamin B_{12} and this figure was higher in those children who had consumed a macrobiotic diet during their entire lifetime. In general, the children were relatively short in stature and low in weight, and decreased stature was associated with low vitamin B_{12} status. It is likely, however, that these children were also deficient in other nutrients that influence growth.

Infants and young children require a well-balanced diet to provide essential energy and nutrients for growth and development (see Chapters 2 and 3 for nutritional requirements) and very restricted diets are not advisable. Macrobiotic diets do not provide adequate energy and protein for infants and young children and if they are following this type of regimen, dietary assessment should be carried out and specific advice given. An infant soya formula should be recommended and supplements given where necessary (see Chapter 2 for information on infant soya formulae).

References

Francis D (1986) *Nutrition for Children*. Oxford, Blackwell Scientific Publications.

Miller DR et al. (1991) Vitamin B_{12} status in a macrobiotic community. *American Journal of Clinical Nutrition* **53,** 524–9.

Sams C (1972) *About Macrobiotics — The Way of Eating*. London, Thorsons.

Further reading

Hill SE (1990) *More than Rice and Peas*. Guidelines to improve food provision for black and ethnic minorities in Britain. London, Food Commission.

Langley G (1988) *Vegan Nutrition — A Survey of Research*. Oxford, Vegan Society.

Thomas B (1988) *Manual of Dietetic Practice*. Oxford, Blackwell Scientific Publications.

7

Vegetarianism and food beliefs

Key points

1. Types of vegetarian diets range from simply avoiding red meat through to more restrictive diets.

2. In an omnivorous diet, animal foods normally provide substantial amounts of food energy, protein, calcium, iron, zinc, vitamins A, D and B_{12}. A well-planned and varied vegetarian diet will provide adequate energy and nutrients but problems can arise if those foods excluded are not replaced by suitable alternatives in terms of the nutrients they supply.

3. Many teenagers are adopting a vegetarian style of eating. Special attention should be given to the iron intake of girls.

4. A vegetarian diet that maintains good health in adulthood may not necessarily be appropriate for infants and young children.

Prevalence of vegetarianism

Research carried out by Gallup in 1993 on behalf of the Realeat Company (makers of vegetarian foods such as the Vegeburger) indicated that 4.3% of the population aged 16 and over do not eat meat and fish, showing an increase since the 1990 Realeat survey of 16%. This represents a total of two and a half million people. Realeat predicts that by the turn of the century there could be five million vegetarians and a total of 10 million non-meat eaters in Great Britain.

Young women are leading the way in the trend towards vegetarianism with 13.3% of 16–24 year old women, three times the national average, being vegetarian. However, vegetarianism is also increasing in men. The Realeat survey (1993) showed that there was a 48% increase, since 1990, in the number of 25–34 year old men who are vegetarian, and an increase in the 35–44 year old age group of 59%.

In previous Realeat surveys, which began in 1984, the higher socio-economic groups were more likely to be vegetarian and did not eat meat. However, in the latest survey (1993) the most radical changes were apparent in the C2, D and E social groups.

Types of vegetarian diets

The term 'vegetarian' is used to describe a whole range of diets (Table 7.1).

Implications for health

Variations in strictness of vegetarianism (Table 7.1) are great and are largely dependent on the person's beliefs and reasons for adopting vegetarianism. This may be for a variety of personal, philosophical, ecological and economic reasons. Some understanding of these reasons is important when considering nutritional status.

To ensure a nutritionally balanced diet a variety of foods should be selected from the four main food groups (see Appendix 1 and Part 1, page 31).

Protein

Complementary combinations of protein-containing foods include:

- pulses/rice — bean casserole and rice, dhal and rice

Table 7.1 *Types of vegetarian diets*

Term	Description
'Semi' or 'demi' vegetarian	Exclusion of red meat or all meat, but fish and other animal products are still consumed; some people also exclude poultry
Lacto-ovo-vegetarian	Exclusion of all meat, fish and poultry; milk, milk products and eggs are still consumed
Lacto-vegetarian	Exclusion of all meat, fish, poultry and eggs; milk and milk products are still consumed
Vegan	Exclusion of all foods of animal origin; diets comprise vegetables, vegetable oils, cereals, pulses such as beans and lentils, nuts, fruit and seeds
Fruitarian	Exclusion of all foods of animal origin as well as pulses and cereals. Diets mainly comprise raw and dried fruit, nuts, honey and olive oil. People following this type of eating pattern are at great risk of nutritional deficiency; their diets require vitamin and mineral supplementation
Macrobiotic — sometimes referred to as Zen Macrobiotic diet (see Chapter 6)	The diet progresses through a series of levels, gradually eliminating all animal produce, fruit and vegetables and leading to a restricted diet of cereal (brown rice) only. Fluids are also severely restricted. Children are particularly at risk of nutritional deficiency

- pulses/cereal — baked beans on toast
- nuts/cereal — peanut butter sandwich.

Plant foods have a low concentration of one or more essential amino acids. However, if proteins from different plant sources are eaten together (or at least over a day), the amino acid profiles of the plant proteins will complement each other. Deficits in amino acids in any one plant protein will be compensated for by the amino acids in another.

Minerals

Frank deficiencies of minerals are not widespread in vegetarian populations. This may be due to increased intestinal absorption of nutrients and/or because wise food choices are made. However, some people may be having suboptimal intakes of some minerals, especially those who have recently changed to a vegetarian regimen and may not be well informed about good food choices, or those 'new' vegetarians whose bodies have not had time to adapt to the poorer bioavailability of some nutrients (see below). Both plant and animal sources of minerals are given in Table 7.2.

Calcium
Vegetarians who consume milk and milk products are likely to have adequate intakes of calcium. Vegans may be having below optimal intakes of calcium as relatively few other foods contain large amounts, and the bioavailability of calcium from plant sources may be greatly reduced by fibre, phytate and/or oxalate (Heaney et al., 1988; British Nutrition Foundation, 1989). These substances can form complexes with the calcium which are insoluble and cannot be absorbed.

Iron
Much of the absorbable iron in omnivore diets comes from the consumption of red meat and offal, and the haem iron from these sources is particularly well absorbed. Iron from non-haem sources such as eggs, cereal

Table 7.2 *Animal and plant sources of vitamins and minerals*

Nutrient	Animal sources	Plant sources
Protein	Meat, poultry, fish, eggs, milk, cheese, yogurt	Soya protein, pulses, bread, grains, seeds, potatoes
Calcium	Milk, cheese, yogurt, tinned sardines, and salmon including the bones (the soft bones should not be discarded)	Fortified soya milk, tofu, seeds (e.g. sesame seeds), green leafy vegetables (e.g. spring greens), nuts (e.g. almonds), bread (especially white bread), dried fruit (e.g. apricots)
Iron	Liver, red meat, chicken, fish, eggs (non-haem iron)	Fortified breakfast cereals (the label should be checked to see if iron has been added), bread, pulses (e.g. soya beans), green vegetables, dried fruits (e.g. apricots), nuts, plain chocolate
Vitamin A	Liver, butter, whole milk, cheese	Yellow/orange vegetables* (e.g. carrots) and dark green leafy ones (e.g. parsley, watercress), yellow/orange fruit (e.g. mangoes, and apricots — fresh or dried), fortified margarine, sweet potato
Vitamin B$_{12}$	Liver, meat, poultry, fish, milk and milk products, eggs	Fortified products (e.g. soya milk), some margarines (Pure, Suma), textured vegetable protein products, and some infant foods
Vitamin D	Oily fish, whole milk and its products, eggs	Fortified margarine, fortified breakfast cereals (the label should be checked to see if vitamin D has been added)

*In vegetables and fruit, vitamin A is in the form of carotenoids, e.g. beta-carotene.

foods, potatoes, green vegetables, nuts and pulses is less well absorbed. The presence of vitamin C from fruit, fruit juices and vegetables will enhance the absorption of non-haem iron; for example, having an iron-fortified breakfast cereal and a glass of orange juice at the same meal. However, tea, coffee (because of tannins) and components of non-starch polysaccharides such as phytate and oxalates reduce iron absorption.

Meeting physiological iron requirements in childhood and adolescence may be a problem for vegetarians and demands careful dietary planning. The reference nutrient intake (see Part 1, Chapter 2) for iron for teenage girls is 14.8 mg per day. However, the intakes of two-thirds of female British teenagers is below

12 mg per day, and a larger number have intakes below 14.8 mg per day. Although this low intake does not imply deficiency, some of these girls, especially those with high menstrual losses, may not be meeting their individual needs for iron and could be at risk of iron deficiency and iron deficiency anaemia. Potential problems may arise if anaemia which developed during the teenage years persists into childbearing years threatening the long-term health of their offspring (Godfrey et al., 1991).

In a study carried out by Nelson and colleagues (1993), which investigated the level of iron deficiency and iron deficiency anaemia in a group of apparently healthy 12–14 year old white schoolchildren, 10.5% of girls were anaemic, 4% had low iron stores (indicated by low ferritin levels) and 16% had borderline iron stores. Anaemia was three times more common in vegetarians than omnivores (25% against 9%), and in girls who had tried to lose weight in the last year compared with those who had not (23% versus 7%).

It is therefore important that dietary sources of iron (Table 7.2) are eaten daily and the bioavailability of the iron in those particular foods is considered — the inclusion of a food source of vitamin C and exclusion of tea at a meal containing non-haem iron (for example in green vegetables and wholegrain cereals).

Zinc

Foods considered to be the most abundant sources of this mineral include meat, poultry, dairy products, bread and other cereal products, and seafood. If many of these foods are excluded, dietary intake may be low but it is thought that adaptation to the diet might occur with time, resulting in an increase in the proportion of zinc absorbed from the intestine.

Vitamins

Most vitamins can be provided by foods of plant origin. However, vitamin B_{12} is found only in foods of animal origin, and there are few dietary sources of vitamin D (Table 7.2).

Vitamin B_{12}

It is essential that vegans, and other people who avoid all animal foods, include a source of vitamin B_{12} in their diet, either as a supplement (usually in tablet form) or as fortified foods (Table 7.2).

Fermented products, such as tempeh and miso (obtained from fermented soya beans), and yeast extracts contain substances which are similar chemically to vitamin B_{12} but do not have the biological activity of the vitamin. Therefore, these foods cannot be regarded as rich in this vitamin (Herbert, 1988) and should not be recommended as a suitable source. In fact, it has been suggested that these substances compete with vitamin B_{12}

for absorption and a high intake may precipitate a vitamin B_{12} deficiency.

Vitamin D

Although rare in Caucasians in Britain, low vitamin D status has been reported among the Asian population, particularly among children, adolescents and women (James et al., 1985; Finch, 1992; Iqbal et al., 1994), many of whom are vegetarian. Prolonged deficiency of vitamin D results in rickets in children and osteomalacia in adults. A combination of factors may be associated with low vitamin D status (Henderson et al., 1987; Clements, 1989) including:

- **low exposure to sunlight:** this may be due to seclusion or strict dress codes limiting vitamin D synthesis in the skin. Ultra violet light is only of the correct wavelength for vitamin D synthesis between about March and October. In addition, pigments in the skin are thought to filter out some of the ultra violet light, and it has been suggested that Asians may have a defective pathway in the conversion of the inactive form of vitamin D to the active form.

- **type of vegetarian diet:** vitamin D is found naturally in only a few foods, all of which are of animal origin, for example oily fish such as mackerel and sardines, eggs, whole milk and its products. Some breakfast cereals and all margarines (required by law in the UK to contain vitamin D) are fortified with vitamin D.

Those who receive little exposure to the sun particularly need to rely more on dietary sources, and it is recommended that Asian children and women take a vitamin D supplement in tablet form (DH, 1991), to prevent the development of rickets and osteomalacia. An adequate intake of calcium is also important in bone development (Table 7.2).

Vegetarian diets and children

A vegetarian diet that keeps adults in good health is not necessarily appropriate for infants and young children, as this is a time of rapid growth and development when a good

Table 7.3 *Weaning foods for vegan diets*[*]

Energy and nutrients	Food	Additional information
Energy	Nut butters[a], sunflower/sesame seed spread (tahini), fortified margarines, oils, avocado	Nuts and seeds should be very finely ground or made into smooth paste as babies can choke on whole or even finely chopped nuts and seeds
Protein	Puréed pulses, puréed cereal,[a] nut butters,[a] potato	It is important to combine different protein sources to provide essential amino acids
Calcium	Puréed cereals[a] — millet, puréed pulses, nut butters,[a] sesame seed spread (tahini), hard water	The bioavailability of calcium from plant sources may be reduced by fibre, phytate and/or oxalate
Vitamin A	Puréed carrots and green leafy vegetables, puréed fruit — apricot, peach, nectarine, pineapple	In vegetables and fruit, vitamin A is in the form of carotenoids, e.g. beta-carotene
Iron	Puréed pulses — especially soya beans, puréed cereals,[a] puréed dark green leafy vegetables, dried fruit soaked and puréed, molasses and black treacle,[b] fortified infant foods	The presence of foods containing vitamin C **at the same meal** is important to aid absorption of iron
Zinc	Puréed cereals,[a] nut butters[a]	
Vitamin B group	Puréed cereal[a] (whole grain), puréed vegetables, fortified infant foods	
Vitamin B$_{12}$	Fortified infant food, fortified breakfast cereals,[a] fortified TVP, fortified yeast extracts[c]	Yeast extracts are too salty for children under six months of age. Very small quantities can be included after this age
Vitamin C	Puréed fruit and vegetables: citrus fruit,[a] berry fruit, green leafy vegetables (lightly cooked), bean sprouts, red and green peppers, radish, sorrel, new potatoes	Fruit juices should ideally be provided with meals only, and not given in a bottle but in a cup (see Chapters 2 and 13)
Vitamin D	Fortified margarines, fortified infant food	A major source of vitamin D for vegan children is sunlight but care must be taken to avoid over-exposure

[*]For vegan infants, infant formula based on soya protein contains all these nutrients.
[a]Wheat-based foods, nut butters and citrus fruit may cause allergic reactions in susceptible infants (see Chapter 2).
[b]May give a taste for sweet things, leading to problems with teeth and weight later.
[c]A baby's kidneys, being immature, cannot readily excrete large amounts of salt.

supply of energy and nutrients is particularly important (Sanders, 1988; O'Connell et al., 1989). Diets that are low in energy and fat and high in bulk may pose a nutritional risk for children when stomach capacity is limited (Pugliese et al., 1987). In addition, the quality of the adults' diets will naturally influence the early choices made by their children. If processed foods such as vegeburgers and vegebangers make up the main part of the family's diet, this may well be reflected in the diets of young children. Advice on construction of a good vegetarian regimen is essential during the antenatal period, such as at family planning clinics or antenatal classes.

The presence of milk and milk products and perhaps eggs in a child's vegetarian diet is likely to ensure that adequate amounts of calcium, vitamin B_{12}, vitamin D and riboflavin are supplied. These nutrients may need supplementation in a vegan diet. A wide range of foods should be given daily following the same guidelines as for adults (Chapters 2 and 3, and Part 1, Chapters 5 and 9) with an adequate supply of energy and nutrient-dense foods such as milk, cheese, margarine and nut butters (whole nuts should not be given to children under five years of age). One pint of cows' milk or its equivalent in yogurt or rennet-free cheese, or a fortified soya milk should be consumed daily.

Vegan diets are **not** recommended during the weaning period. However, if such a regimen is followed, weaning should follow the same principles as for non-vegan babies (see Chapter 2), and at least a pint per day of infant soya formula should be consumed. Table 7.3 shows foods which may be suitable for weaning onto a vegan diet. In addition, some commercial weaning foods may be suitable. It is recommended that all vegan children under five years of age should receive supplements of vitamin drops containing vitamins A, C and D. Foods fortified with vitamin B_{12} should be included in the diet and, if necessary, a vitamin B_{12} supplement (usually in tablet form).

References

British Nutrition Foundation (1989) *Calcium. Report of the British Nutrition Foundation's Task Force.* London, BNF.

Clements MR (1989) The problem of rickets in UK Asians. *Journal of Human Nutrition and Dietetics* **2,** 105–16.

Department of Health, Committee on Medical Aspects of Food Policy (1991) *Dietary Reference Values for Food Energy and Nutrients for the United Kingdom. Report on Health and Social Subjects 41.* London, HMSO.

Finch PJ (1992) Blunted seasonal variation in serum 2-hydroxy vitamin D and increased risk of osteomalacia in vegetarian London Asians. *European Journal of Clinical Nutrition* **46,** 509–15.

Godfrey KM et al. (1991) The effect of maternal anaemia and iron deficiency on the ratio of fetal weight to placental weight. *British Journal of Obstetrics and Gynaecology* **98,** 167–79.

Heaney RP et al. (1988) Calcium absorbability from spinach. *American Journal of Clinical Nutrition* **47,** 707–9.

Henderson JB et al. (1987) The importance of limited exposure to ultraviolet radiation and dietary factors on the aetiology of Asian rickets: a risk factor model. *Quarterly Journal of Medicine* **63,** 413–25.

Herbert V (1988) Vitamin B_{12}: plant sources, requirements, and assay. *American Journal of Clinical Nutrition* **48,** 852–8.

Iqbal SJ et al. (1994) Evidence of continuing 'deprivational' vitamin D deficiency in Asians in the UK. *Journal of Human Nutrition and Dietetics* **7,** 47–52.

James JA et al. (1985) Screening Rastafarian children for nutritional rickets. *British Medical Journal* **290,** 899.

Nelson M et al. (1993) Haemoglobin, ferritin and iron intakes in British children aged 12–14 years: a preliminary investigation. *British Journal of Nutrition* **70,** 147–55.

O'Connell JM et al. (1989) Growth of vegetarian children: The Farm Study. *Paediatrics* **84,** 475–81.

Pugliese MT et al. (1987) Parental health beliefs as a cause of failure to thrive. *Paediatrics* **80,** 175–82.

Realeat (1990) *Changing Attitudes to Meat Consumption.* London, Realeat.

Realeat (1993) *Changing Attitudes to Meat Consumption.* London, Realeat.

Sanders TAB (1988) Growth and development of British vegan children. *American Journal of Clinical Nutrition* **48,** 822–5.

Further reading

National Dairy Council (1995) *Nutrition and Teenagers. Fact File 5 (revised).* London, NDC.

8

Low income families

Key points

1. Ill health is more prevalent among those living on low incomes, and mortality from diseases such as coronary heart disease is also greater. It has been suggested recently that this susceptibility to heart disease may be determined by maternal health and by nutrition *in utero* and during the first year of life.

2. Although eating a healthy diet is possible on a low income, in reality those living on a low income typically consume fewer of the foods regarded as 'healthy' and their diet is often less varied.

3. Provision of nutrition education for families on a low income poses particular problems as improving dietary habits may be low on a list of competing priorities faced by the family. Nevertheless, there is often a willingness to change and an awareness of what changes are required, which can be built upon.

4. A variety of obstacles and barriers to change exacerbate the difficulties faced by those on low income who attempt to provide a healthier diet for their family. These obstacles are discussed.

5. The primary health care team can be a focus and an instrument of social change. Practical ideas are given for improving diets at low cost.

Definitions of a 'poverty line' vary but two definitions sometimes used are when the proportion of the net family income spent on food is above 25% or above 30%. Those whose level of income may influence their ability to provide a varied diet for themselves or their dependants include:

- students
- pensioners
- those on benefits
- those in work but on very low incomes
- single parents
- those with a low residual income per family (i.e. moderate income but large family).

A change in family circumstances may result in the amount of money coming into the household suddenly falling or outgoings rising. This, too, can affect ability to provide an adequate and varied diet for the family.

Low income and health

In 1980, the Black Report indicated that ill health was more prevalent among people with low incomes and that they were more likely to die prematurely (DHSS, 1980). A report by Davey Smith et al. (1990) suggested that ten years on, social class differences in mortality appeared to be widening and that these differences exist for health during life. Such health inequalities have been shown in all countries that collect relevant data.

Much ill health in later life is thought to be preventable provided that appropriate action is taken in childhood to eliminate the adverse conditions known to affect future health. In their report *Give us a Chance*, the Child Poverty Action Group, the Health Visitors' Association and the Save the Children Fund point to the right of children to the best opportunities to maximize their health potential (Seymour, 1992). However, they believe that children's health is also influenced by the health of their parents, especially the mother; and improving the parents' health will therefore improve the health of the child.

The report of the Social Security Select Committee on distribution of income, published in 1991, revealed that between 1979 and 1988 the number of people living on incomes below half the national average, after housing costs, increased from 4.9 million to 11.8 million (SSSC, 1991; Seymour, 1992). Within this group, children were disproportionately represented: in 1979, 1.6 million children lived in households in this category and by 1988 the figure had risen to 3.01 million.

The Black Report offers various explanations for the inequalities in health associated with social class (DHSS, 1980). These explanations tend to emphasize those hazards which are inherent in society, and to which those with low incomes and low levels of opportunity are inevitably exposed. The health-damaging effects of physico-chemical exposures in certain occupations have long been recognized (Hunter, 1955) and recent research has shown the importance of income (Wilkinson, 1989), psychosocial factors (Marmot and Theorell, 1989), poor quality or damp housing (Martin et al., 1987) and employment status (Moser et al., 1990).

There is also a possibility that deprivation in early life can affect the subsequent health of adults. Barker and colleagues have proposed that cardiovascular and respiratory diseases may have their origins in adverse conditions in early childhood. Recently, they have linked the ratio of birth weight to placental weight with risk of subsequent hypertension in adulthood (Barker et al., 1990), low birth weight and weight gain in the first year with increased risk of non-insulin dependent diabetes later in life (Hales et al., 1991), and thinness and small head circumference at birth to increased risk of death from cardiovascular disease in adulthood (Barker et al., 1993). (See Chapter 10.)

Low income and diet

In general, there are no data available to indicate that those with low incomes suffer specific nutritional deficiencies. However, some recent work has shown cases of low iron status and iron deficiency anaemia among infants and preschool children (Aukett et al., 1986; James et al., 1989; Marder et al., 1990; Mills, 1990) and this is particularly prevalent among immigrant children and those living in families with low income (see Chapters 2 and 3).

There has been considerable interest in the possibility that health-related behaviour — particularly cigarette smoking, diet and lack of exercise — results in inequalities of health. A major variation in diet is the lower intakes of fruit and vegetables among families living on a low income (for other differences, see page 84). Intakes of vitamin C, carotenoids and fibre are consequently less in lower social classes, and the sodium to potassium ratio is higher.

The first two of these nutrients are antioxidants, important in protecting the body against harmful free radicals. These small molecules are now thought to be instrumental in diseases such as cancer and heart disease. In addition, intake of trans fatty acids (see Chapter 10) are likely to be greater through an increased intake of the cheaper margarines made from hydrogenated vegetable oils.

Coupled with these dietary differences, and in common with other income groups, those on low income often have high levels of fat, sugar and salt in their diets. Consequently, in order to meet dietary targets, those living on a low income need to make the same dietary changes as other sectors of the population, but are likely to face greater obstacles in doing so (see page 83). However, some would argue that specific educational messages about nutrition are needed for those in poverty because micronutrient intakes may be compromised alongside macronutrient intakes. This is currently under consideration by a Health of the Nation project team (see page 89).

However, before nutrition issues can be tackled, it is often necessary to address other problems associated with the circumstances of low income families including depression and low self-esteem. These problems can override concern about food (see page 84).

Furthermore, being poor demands greater creativity in the context of the skills needed to provide a healthy diet for the family. There is also a need for considerable commitment to overcome the various barriers which are encountered regularly.

Low income and health promotion

Health promotion messages often take insufficient account of the social and economic circumstances in which people find themselves, and the limited choices open to them. As a result people, particularly women, are made to feel inadequate because it is implied they are bad managers of the family budget or they simply do not care enough about how they feed their families.

In reality, however, a number of studies now show that women operating under the constraints of a very low budget purchase food wisely and frequently succeed in meeting the nutrient and energy needs of those they care for, though this is sometimes at considerable personal cost (Women's Information Network, 1988; HVA Nutrifax, 1989; Price and Sephton, 1991). Evidence exists that mothers often cut back or go without food so that the children and their partner get sufficient (Craig et al., 1990). However, in achieving this objective, the diets though adequate are often lacking in variety and rely heavily on a small number of staple foods such as bread and potatoes. People living in such circumstances may need to be reassured that diets of this nature can be nutritionally adequate, though they may not meet their dietary aspirations and personal perception of a 'good' diet.

Cutting back on food purchase is perhaps inevitable as food remains the single biggest item with which families can juggle the family budget when fixed costs such as rent, fuel and Council Tax need to be met. Because of low income, poor families devote a much higher proportion of their expenditure to basic necessities such as food. Nevertheless, people with low incomes tend to buy their food more efficiently in nutritional terms and in terms of value for money than more affluent families (Nelson and Peploe, 1990). This trend is particularly marked for foods such as bread, fats, potatoes and sugar.

Barriers to change and motivating factors

One of the main objectives of nutrition education has been to improve people's nutritional knowledge, on the assumption that people eat 'less healthy' food through lack of knowledge. However, a number of surveys have shown that while there is confusion on some issues, general levels of knowledge about food and health are high across all social classes. Knowledge is not the main barrier to change. The National Food Survey indicates that consumption of healthy food (those foods for which increased consumption is encouraged in current healthy eating guidelines, such as those described by HEA et al., 1990) occurs to some extent across all income groups (MAFF, 1992a). One report indicated that for the lower income groups basic nutrition, satisfying appetite and day-to-day welfare were more central to the concept of eating than long-term health issues (HEA, 1989).

The main barriers to change (NDC/MORI, 1992 a, b) seem to be:

- taste
- family preferences
- poor cooking facilities
- concerns about wastage when experimenting with new foods
- cost.

Other important barriers, for some at least, are:

- difficulties regarding access to and local availability of healthier food choices at a reasonable price — corner shops are usually more expensive than supermarkets and offer a limited choice

- inability to cook and so reliance on familiar items through lack of confidence and because a failed 'experiment' can prove very costly and leave the family hungry

- inability to store food at home

- low self-esteem — a change from long-standing dietary habits requires additional forethought and planning, together with considerable commitment which may not come easily to those who are socially deprived

- false belief that a healthy diet is already being consumed.

It has also been assumed that in order to motivate change, there should be a focus on long-term health risks associated with consuming a less healthy diet. However, this approach requires people to take a long-term view of their health. Particularly among those living on low incomes, there are frequently more pressing short-term considerations such as unemployment or poor housing.

Although a healthy diet which meets dietary reference values can be put together for a relatively low cost, it will inevitably be considerably different from the sort of diet currently eaten by most people in the UK. In particular, the diet is likely to be less varied and heavily reliant on staple foods.

A number of studies have suggested that although guidance on combinations of foods which meet the dietary guidelines at low cost can be produced, subgroups of the population are unable to afford a healthy diet which is based on adjustments to the typical British diet (Cole Hamilton and Lang, 1986; Hanes and de Looy, 1987; Cade and Booth, 1990).

So, when money is tight, changing to a healthier diet is not always an easy step; 'healthier' options which are direct substitutes for foods previously eaten are often more expensive, and mothers may feel that they cannot afford to experiment or to risk the unfamiliar food being wasted and the family being dissatisfied and hungry. In addition, food is not simply a fuel. The ideal of food being enjoyable is often forgotten during this process of communicating information about healthy eating, particularly when people are being encouraged to switch to unfamiliar

'healthier' options. Furthermore, associated with food and eating are a variety of social and religious attitudes and beliefs which should not be ignored (see Chapter 6).

Nutrition education programmes are more likely to be successful if they are built around the participants' current knowledge and skills, and take full account of their concerns, beliefs and circumstances, perhaps addressing lack of confidence in cooking skills and providing opportunities for tasting and cooking healthy meals using cheap, readily available ingredients. It is essential that the participants are in control of the learning process and are involved in the development of the project at all stages. A community development approach also has the potential to modify the environment within which the participants live, by looking at ways to influence the foods available cheaply in local shops, and by setting up food co-operatives and bulk-buying schemes. In the longer term, it may be possible for those involved in such projects to influence the teaching of food-related topics in local schools, so as to improve knowledge of nutrition and food preparation (see page 89).

Concerns about food are often a low priority in the lives of people surviving on a very low income in very poor housing in a deprived area, and nutrition education must be viewed against a background of competing priorities. What might seem a pressing priority for health workers may be low down the list of the priorities determined by the family.

Constructing a healthy diet

The 1991 and subsequent National Food Surveys indicated that although families with low income spend less on food, they buy more basic staples such as bread, flour, potatoes, eggs, tea and sugar (MAFF, 1992a).

People with low incomes are also more likely to eat very small amounts of vegetables and fruit; small amounts of fruit juice; white bread rather than wholemeal; fatty meats and meat products instead of lean meat; food that is fried, especially in hard fats; and more sugar and preserves than those who are better off. Consequently, the nutritional value and balance of the diet is affected. In particular, intake of vitamin C is usually lower in larger and poorer families (MAFF, 1992a).

A healthy balanced diet contains a large proportion of cereal food, starchy vegetables, other vegetables and fruit, and moderate amounts of foods such as lean meat, fish and dairy produce (see Appendix 1 and Part 1, page 31). Biscuits and confectionery may be cheaper in terms of calories per pound (£1), but they provide fewer essential nutrients.

A number of studies indicate that the cost of a diet which takes into account social factors, and is in line with current dietary advice and individual preferences, can be significantly more than the amount of money most people with low incomes have to spend on food (Hanes and de Looy, 1987; Stitt, 1990).

The following are some ideas for anyone wishing to improve the quality of their diet while watching costs (Nelson and Peploe, 1990):

- Increase potato consumption and replace half the white bread consumed by wholemeal. Eat more pasta and rice.

- Use only small amounts of fat in cooking and replace the calories with extra bread (particularly wholemeal), rice or pasta.

- Spread butter or margarine thinly on thicker slices of bread.

- Fruit and vegetables that are in season are often cheaper. Buy in small quantities to avoid having to store them and risk them going off. Although bruised or damaged fruit and vegetables may be cheaper, they deteriorate quickly and the vitamin content is a little lower.

- Frozen vegetables are a useful alternative if freezer space is available.

- Add extra pulses and vegetables to meals such as shepherds pie to make the meat go further.

- Cook mince without adding fat and drain off any fat after cooking. Meat does not have to be expensive to be nutritious — lean mince is as good a source of iron as best steak.

- Use plain yogurt or fromage frais instead of packet toppings.

- Use small amounts of strong cheese in cooking rather than larger amounts of mild cheese. Cheese can be grated for salads or sandwiches to make it go further.

- Eat fewer convenience foods with relatively poor nutritional value such as instant meals in pots, sweet dessert mixes, sweet drinks, confectionery, packet snack foods and sweet biscuits.

- When using the oven, cook a few items at one time to save fuel, for example jacket potatoes, a casserole and a milk pudding. Bake jacket potatoes with a metal skewer through them as they will cook more quickly.

- Use left-overs in another meal, but store them carefully (see Appendix 2).

Dissemination of recipes developed locally using readily available and economical ingredients, for example through 'cook and eat' sessions, is often a useful practice.

For general information on healthy eating, see Part 1, and for further suggestions and fuel saving ideas, see "Eating Well on a Budget", part of a free pack from the National Dairy Council (1993), which is suitable for group work.

Work carried out by MAFF (1992b), utilizing the National Food Survey data, has indicated that an adequate diet, meeting the dietary reference values (DH, 1991) could be purchased in 1992 for £10.00 per person per week. This was called the 'low cost' diet. For comparison, Table 8.1 shows the average weekly expenditure per head on food at the time when the calculations were made. This serves to emphasize the importance of household food in the overall food bill, particularly for low income families. Interestingly,

Table 8.1 *Expenditure on food* in relation to available income*

Type of household	Per capita weekly expenditure on food consumed within the home	Total per capita weekly expenditure on food, including sweets, alcohol and meals out
Average	£13.84	£22.15
Households with a total of less than £60 to spend per week	£13.71	£17.27
Households with a total of more than £800 to spend per week	£17.19	£34.45

*This information is taken from the National Food Survey, conducted annually by the Ministry of Agriculture, Fisheries and Food. It relates to the 1991 survey.
Source: MAFF (1992b).

expenditure on food per head is influenced more by the number of people in the household than by income.

The £10.00 'low cost' diet is a theoretical diet designed to meet the dietary reference values. For acceptability it was based on current British eating patterns but, perhaps inevitably because of cost implications, focuses on increased intakes of cheaper and filling (staple) foods, coupled with reductions in some foods of animal origin.

In order to meet the dietary guidelines for energy and nutrients **at low cost**, MAFF calculated that quite considerable changes to the current British diet would be needed. For instance, intakes of foods such as meat, meat products, fish, cheese and eggs would need to fall. MAFF proposed that intake of milk could remain at current levels, as could intakes of spreading and cooking fats. To meet the target of £10.00, fresh fruit and vegetable consumption would remain at current levels, but intakes of fruit products and other types of vegetables (processed and frozen) and tinned beans would need to rise considerably to meet nutrient needs. Intakes of staples such as bread, potatoes and other cereals (including breakfast cereals) would need to rise too. Finally they proposed the need for a reduction in consumption of cakes, buns and pastries, but allowed a small increase in sugar consumption.

It has to be questioned whether those living on a low income would be prepared to make changes such as these which, because of the restrictions on cost, are considerably greater in some cases than would be needed by those with more money to spend on food and are also far greater than the extent of change which has been achieved so far as a result of nutrition education initiatives.

These changes in diet might also be considered as setting those on a low income as a race apart because several of the recommended changes run counter to the advice on healthy eating currently offered to the general population.

Out of necessity, calculations of this nature do not take account of family composition. It should not be assumed, though, that food and the nutrients it contains are usually distributed equally among family members (see page 83).

To be of any use to the public, dietary guidelines and the subsequent need for dietary changes need to be translated into practical and user-friendly advice for individuals and families to follow. A collaborative project under the auspices of Health of the Nation orchestrated by the Department of Health, Health Education Authority and MAFF has taken one major step down this route by developing a Food Selection Guide, "The Balance of Good Health" (see Appendix 1).

The purpose of this food grouping system is to help people understand the relative importance of the various groups of foods available to us. As discussed in Part 1, we regularly need to eat foods from the milk group of foods and from the meat and alternatives foods, but we should consume a greater proportion of our food from the fruit and vegetables group and the bread and cereals group. For example, most people will benefit from eating more fruit and vegetables and should aim for about five servings daily from this group. On the other hand, two to three servings from the milk and milk products group will be adequate for most people except those with very high calcium needs. More detailed information can be found in Part 1 on what might constitute a serving and how the dietary changes implicated by the Food Selection Guide might be brought about (see Part 1, Chapter 9).

Purchasing food

The Health Education Authority's report on healthy eating in low income groups shows that participants in the study tended to adopt a 'tunnel vision' approach to shopping, only allowing themselves to look for familiar items. Food choice depended on acceptability to the family, with little experimentation in order to prevent wastage (HEA, 1989).

Purchasing nutritious food of good quality in economic quantities for a family requires planning, transport and suitable storage space at home. The following are useful suggestions when money is tight:

- Shopping might be shared with friends and costs split.

- Shared transport for shopping trips is cheaper.

- Forward planning will prevent the need for emergency buys, which can be more expensive.

- Meat bought from the butcher can be cut to requirement rather than pre-packaged.

This will sometimes be cheaper.

- Some goods are reduced in price late in the day or at weekends.

- Compare prices — 'own brands' may sometimes be cheaper. Large bargain packs can be shared with a friend or neighbour.

Take-away and convenience foods

In many circumstances, such as where transport is difficult or for those living in bed and breakfast accommodation where there are no cooking facilities, take-away food can sometimes be a more practical option.

The best café and fast foods are those which do not contain a lot of fat or sugar and are rich in essential nutrients. Examples of healthier convenience and take-away foods include:

- sandwiches — bread, pitta or large rolls (preferably wholemeal) filled with meat (e.g. roast chicken, beef, lamb, ham), cheese or canned fish (e.g. tuna, sardines, mackerel) **and** salad

- filled jacket potatoes

- shish kebabs and salad

- plain burger in brown bun and salad

- fruit

- yogurt

- breakfast cereals

- milk

- fruit juice.

Regardless of what the main meal comprises, it is important to include some salad, vegetables or fruit with the meal, for example fish and chips with peas, salad or baked beans (see Part 1). A good rule of thumb is to include at least one item from each of the cereal and fruit/vegetables groups at each meal, and to include one item from the meat and alternatives group and the milk and milk products group at two meals each day.

James, a Bristol general practitioner, and his practice team have shown in a small study that one-to-one counselling of mothers living in poor circumstances can result in improved diet for them and their children (James et al., 1992). This project was the impetus for production of a pack for health professionals working with low income families, available free of charge from the National Dairy Council (1993).

Ethnic minorities

A significant proportion of the people living on low income in Britain are from ethnic minorities and may need advice tailored specifically to their needs, particularly if their diet is largely traditional. Information on the broad dietary practices of some ethnic minority groups can be found in Chapter 6. Below are some ideas on how these practices can be integrated with healthy eating guidelines for three ethnic groups (NDC, 1993).

The Asian community

It is not possible to make an Asian meal without adding any fat, and so the normal advice for healthy eating with Western foods is not practical for Asian cookery and needs to be modified. The following advice for 'low fat' cooking methods can be offered:

- Only use very small amounts of fat in cooking; it may help to measure it out.

- Use a pure cooking oil such as rapeseed, olive or sunflower oil; but as these are more expensive than ghee or butter and there may be reluctance to change, re-inforce the message regarding low fat cooking with ghee and tackle the change to unsaturated oil later.

- Cooking with low fat spreads is not successful.

- Avoid adding fat to chapatti dough or prepared chapattis (spreading low fat spread simply makes the cooked chapattis stick together).

- Avoid adding extra fat to food at the table.

Dishes made with pulses are cheap and nutritious but must not be made too thin.

Vegetarians should have pulses daily as they provide protein and iron. Yogurt should be eaten with vegetable dishes to provide extra protein.

Lower fibre chapatti flours tend to be cheaper and so are frequently used. However, high fibre chapattis are often more filling.

A change to brown rice may not be accepted readily. If fibre intake is good, it may not be necessary to advise a change.

In many cases, large quantities of a food are cooked to last the family several days. This practice can reduce the nutrient content because of the need to reheat. Advise that at least one fresh dish is cooked daily. This will also improve variety.

The Afro-Caribbean community

The diets consumed by Afro-Caribbeans in Britain can be high in fat, salt and sugar and appropriate dietary advice may be needed.

Advice to cut down on fat includes:

- cutting down the amount of oil used, for example to fry chicken

- baking some foods that are normally fried, for example dumplings

- reducing the use of saturated oils such as coconut cream/oil and palm oil.

Use more fruit and vegetables, including traditional vegetables such as green bananas, yams, sweet potatoes.

Encourage pulse-based (e.g. rice and peas) and fish-based meals.

Traditionally, sweet foods are not eaten regularly but as people become more affluent, sweet foods are eaten more often. Keep such foods and traditional drinks, for example punch made with sweetened condensed milk, for special occasions.

Advice may be needed about tea and coffee, which is sometimes taken sweetened and with condensed or evaporated milk.

Some traditional dishes use salted meat or fish. Even after soaking, large amounts of salt remain and so these foods should be used sparingly.

Chinese communities

As in many other cultures, moderate increases in affluence can modify a balanced traditional eating pattern and increase consumption of fat and sugar. In attempting to reverse the less desirable trends associated with migration and to promote healthy eating, it is important to be aware of traditional ideas that may cause resistance to ideas commonly advocated in Britain:

- Salads and raw vegetables are rarely eaten.

- A meal is often not considered complete without boiled white rice and hence there will be resistance to brown rice. Wholemeal bread is similarly unpopular.

- Alternatives to fattier meats such as duck are largely acceptable, for example, chicken, fish, vegetarian dishes.

- Although encouraging steaming instead of stir-frying would seem an obvious 'healthy' alternative, steaming is often followed by dressing with oil mixtures.

- Many savoury dishes traditionally include sugar, for example sweet and sour dishes.

- Traditionally, good health depends on a balance of yin and yang. This may need to be taken into consideration (see Chapter 6).

Action by the primary health care team

In Part 1, Chapter 7 the basics of planning a nutrition protocol were discussed. These concepts can readily be applied to planning and implementing a nutrition strategy which facilitates the primary health care team to function as a focus for social change. For example, links can be made with 'neighbourhood centres' in deprived areas, family intervention initiatives such as cook-and-eat sessions can be offered ('hands-on' opportunities to cook and experiment with different ingredients), and food co-operatives can be supported. Other possibilities for action include community cafés and endorsement of activities designed to facilitate social change locally, for example projects dealing with the price or availability of food (anti-poverty projects). Local initiatives often benefit from networking between the voluntary sector and health care personnel, and incorporating industrial, local authority and retail inputs. Examples of contemporary research can be found in Dowler and Rushton (1994).

Each of these approaches has its own constraints and its own set of factors which are likely to improve effectiveness. These are currently under investigation by the Low Income Project Team established under the auspices of the Health of the Nation initiative. A useful briefing paper, produced for consideration by the project team, is to be published (Williams and Dowler, 1995).

Evaluation is an important part of any nutrition strategy and suggestions on how this can be conducted are included in Part 1, Chapter 8.

There is a general need to improve the way the aims and objectives of diet, and low income projects are framed so that the achievements of such initiatives can be evaluated more readily (Williams and Dowler, 1995). Many projects set long-term goals, such as "enabling people to eat more healthily", which are almost impossible to evaluate in the normal time span of a project. Few projects express their activities in terms of operational objectives which allow progress and effectiveness to be measured. However, there are plenty of project-specific activities and outcomes which could be used, for example improving sales of fruit and vegetables from a food co-operative, or usage of recipes from a cookery course.

As well as measuring a project's effectiveness against operational objectives, it is also important to try to evaluate strategic and generic objectives concerned with dietary behaviour. Williams and Dowler (1995) give the example that a project might reach the operational objective of increasing cooking skills but not achieve the overall aim of creating dietary change because of competing priorities and constraints. Dietary change can be measured in terms of nutrient intake, food intake and meal consumption patterns. Some projects also evaluate factors associated with self-esteem and well-being which are not directly related to nutrition, for example value attached to the opportunity to get out of the home and meet others, using food as a focus.

References

Aukett MA et al. (1986) Treatment with iron increases weight gain and psychomotor development. *Archives of Disease in Childhood* **61,** 849–57.

Barker DJP et al. (1990) Fetal and placental size and risk of hypertension in adult life. *British Medical Journal* **301,** 259–62.

Barker DJP et al. (1993) The relation of small head circumference and thinness at birth to death from cardiovascular disease in adult life. *British Medical Journal* **306,** 422–6.

Cade J and Booth S (1990) What can people eat to meet the dietary goals: and how much does it cost? *Journal of Human Nutrition and Dietetics* **3,** 199–207.

Cole Hamilton I and Lang T (1986) *Tightening Belts. Report No. 13.* London, Food Commission.

Craig M et al. (1990) *Poverty and Health. The Legacy of the Social Fund.* London, Save the Children Fund.

Davey Smith G et al. (1990) The Black Report on socio-economic inequalities in health ten years on. *British Medical Journal* **301,** 373–7.

Department of Health, Committee on Medical Aspects of Food Policy (1991) *Dietary Reference Values for Food Energy and Nutrients in the United Kingdom. Report on Health and Social Subjects 41.* London, HMSO.

Department of Health and Social Security (1980) *Inequalities in Health. Report of a Research Working Group.* London, DHSS.

Dowler E and Rushton C (1994) *Diet and Poverty in the UK: Contemporary Research Methods and Current Experience.* London, London School of Hygiene and Tropical Medicine.

Hales CN et al. (1991) Foetal and infant growth and impaired glucose intolerance at age 64. *British Medical Journal* **303,** 1019–22.

Hanes FA and de Looy A (1987) Can I afford the diet? *Human Nutrition: Applied Nutrition* **41A,** 1–12.

Health Education Authority (1989) *Diet, Nutrition and 'Healthy Eating' in Low Income Groups.* London, HEA.

Health Education Authority et al. (1990) *Eight Guidelines for a Healthy Diet.* London, HMSO.

Health Visitors' Association (1989) *Nutrifax.* London, National Dairy Council.

Hunter D (1955) *The Diseases of Occupations.* London, Hodder and Stoughton.

James J et al. (1989) Preventing iron deficiency in preschool children by implementing an educational and screening programme in an inner city practice. *British Medical Journal* **299,** 838–40.

James J et al. (1992) Improving the diet of under-fives in a deprived inner city practice. *Health Trends* **24,** 161–4.

Marder E et al. (1990) Discovering anaemia at child health clinics. *Archives of Disease in Childhood* **65,** 892–4.

Marmot MG and Theorell T (1989) Social class and cardiovascular disease: the contribution of work. *International Journal of Health Services* **18,** 659–74.

Martin CJ et al. (1987) Housing conditions and health. *British Medical Journal* **294,** 1125–7.

Mills AF (1990) Surveillance for anaemia: risk factors in patterns of milk intake. *Archives of Disease in Childhood* **65,** 428–31.

Ministry of Agriculture, Fisheries and Food (1992a) *Household Food Consumption and Expenditure 1991.* London, HMSO.

Ministry of Agriculture, Fisheries and Food, Food Science Division (1992b) The Cost of Alternative Diets. Paper CP(92)9/3. MAFF Consumer Panel Secretariat.

Moser K et al. (1990) Unemployment and mortality. In Goldblatt P (Ed.) *Longitudinal Study: Mortality and Social Organisation.* London, HMSO. pp 81–97.

National Dairy Council and MORI (1992a) *Food and Health: What Does Britain Think?* London, NDC.

National Dairy Council and MORI (1992b) *Food and Health: What Do Health Professionals Think?* London, NDC.

National Dairy Council (1993) *Nutrition and Low Income Families. A Pack for Health Professionals.* London, NDC.

Nelson M and Peploe K (1990) Construction of a modest-but-adequate food budget for households with two adults and one preschool child: a preliminary investigation. *Journal of Human Nutrition and Dietetics* **3,** 121–40.

Price S and Sephton J (1991) *Just Desserts? Influencing Food Choice: Food Behaviour Strategies for Change.* Bradford, Horton Publishing.

Seymour J (1992) *Give us a Chance: Children, Poverty, and the Health of the Nation.* London, Child Poverty Action Group, Health Visitors Association, Save the Children.

Social Security Select Committee (1991) *Low Income Statistics: Households Below Average Income Tables 1988.* London, HMSO.

Stitt S (1990) Poor get little allowance for food. *The Food Magazine*, July/September.

Wilkinson RG (1989) Class mortality differentials, income distribution and trends in poverty 1921–81. *Journal of Social Policy* **18,** 307–35.

Williams C and Dowler E (1995) Identifying successful local projects and initiatives on diet and low income: a review of the issues. In press.

Women's Information Network (1988) *Healthy Eating at What Price?* Belfast, Women's Information Drop In Centre.

Other resources

Avon Look After Your Heart (1993) Eating on a Low Income. Two day courses to help participants develop the necessary skills to give advice and support to those wanting to change their health-related behaviour. (Details: Department of Nutrition and Dietetics, Southmead Hospital, Bristol BS10 5NB.)

Health Education Authority (1988) *Diet, Nutrition and Healthy Eating in Low Income Groups.* London, HEA (0171 383 3833).

Health Education Authority (1991) *Nutrition in Minority Ethnic Groups: Asians and Afro Caribbeans in the United Kingdom.* Briefing Paper. London, HEA.

Health Visitors' Association (1989) *Nutrifax.* Section on: Communicating in partnership. London, National Dairy Council (0171 499 7822).

Hill SE (1990) *More Rice than Peas: Guidelines to Improve Food Provision for Black and Ethnic Minorities in Britain.* London, Food Commission.

Hunt P and Heritage Z (1991) *Access to Healthy Food.* Some women's views on how primary health care workers could help. HEA Primary Health Care Unit, Churchill Hospital, Headington, Oxford OX3 7LJ.

Lawrence B (1991) *How to Feed Your Family for £5.00 a Day.* London, Thorsons.

Malseed J (1990) *Bread without Dough: Understanding Food Poverty.* Bradford, Horton Publishing.

National Children's Home (1991) *Poverty and Nutrition Survey.* London, NCH.

National Community Health Resource (1991) Community Health Initiatives and Food — An Information Pack. London, NCHR (57 Carlton Street, London NW1 1HU Tel: 0171 383 3841).

National Food Alliance (1994) *Food and Low Income.* London, NFA (0171 628 2442).

Rowett Postgraduate Nutrition and Dietetic Centre (1992) When the Money Runs Out. A video and information/training pack. Aberdeen.

9

Nutrition and sport

Key points

1. Good nutrition is important for all sports people, whether they are beginners or seasoned competitors. It forms a key component to any fitness programme, supporting consistent and intensive training.

2. Nutrition is not something that should be considered just before a competition, important game or period of intensive exercise such as a skiing holiday, but rather something that is considered 365 days a year.

3. A healthy diet for sports people should be based on a wide variety of foods which will supply sufficient energy and nutrients.

What to eat

All too often sports people, to satisfy their appetite, rely heavily on foods high in simple carbohydrates in a concentrated form such as confectionery and sugar.

The relative merits of one form of carbohydrate over another, and the number and timing of meals in promoting the repletion of muscle glycogen, is still the focus of much research. In accordance with current advice on healthy eating, starchy carbohydrates ideally should provide half or more of the total energy in the diet. These foods include potatoes, rice, pasta, bread and other cereals including breakfast cereals. These also provide other essential nutrients.

Fat is a concentrated source of energy but since carbohydrate should be supplying the largest proportion of energy in the diet, fat should play a less important role. As a first step, it is preferable to reduce consumption of those fat-containing foods which provide fat and little else of nutritional value (cakes, biscuits, pastries) rather than foods such as meat, eggs and dairy products, which provide other essential nutrients. However, a wide range of low fat dairy products and leaner cuts of meat are now available for those who need to reduce their fat intake still further.

The protein requirement of most athletes is not appreciably greater than that of non-athletes. Most experts recommend a protein intake of 1–2 g per kg body weight per day, which is easy to achieve if the diet is varied and meeting requirements for energy. Only consistent strength training in combination with an adequate diet can increase muscle strength and size. However, attention should be paid to those individuals with low energy intakes and those who exclude all foods of animal origin from their diet (see Chapter 7). The government's report on dietary reference values cautions against high protein intake however, and suggests that intakes more than twice the reference nutrient intake (see Part 1, page 40) should be avoided (DH, 1991).

Energy

Carbohydrate, fat, protein and alcohol are broken down in the body to provide energy (see Table 9.1).

Protein is rarely used by muscles during exercise, except during prolonged exercise when supplies of carbohydrate are short. Alcohol is not metabolized by the working muscles; therefore only carbohydrate (as glucose and glycogen) and fat (as free fatty acids) are important sources of energy for exercising muscles. The proportion of each required will depend on the intensity and

Table 9.1 *Energy value of dietary components*

	Energy yield per gram	
	Kcal	**KJ**
Carbohydrate	3.75	16
Fat	9	37
Protein	4	17
Alcohol	7	29

duration of the activity, as well as the fitness and nutritional status of the individual.

In the first few minutes of exercise and during high intensity exercise (for example sprinting), stored muscle glycogen and circulating blood glucose are the main contributors of energy. During moderate and prolonged exercise, such as jogging, a mixture of carbohydrate and fat is combusted to supply energy (Wootton, 1988).

Following intense exercise, the glycogen stores will be depleted and good nutrition can make its greatest impact by helping recovery between training sessions. The capacity of muscle to refuel is greatest during the first hour after training. Complete refuelling or repletion takes 24 to 48 hours (and longer following very intense exercise) provided the diet contains sufficient starchy carbohydrate-rich foods, such as pasta, rice, potato or cereals (Wootton, 1988).

Vitamins and minerals

There is little hard scientific evidence to suggest that the utilization, destruction or excretion of vitamins is increased with sporting activities, although there have been relatively few well-controlled studies specifically to assess vitamin needs and the nutritional status of people who take part in a lot of sport.

Consuming adequate amounts of iron and calcium is often difficult for many female athletes, particularly those trying to attain a low body weight. Amenorrhoeic women may need additional calcium, possibly as much as 1000 mg to 1500 mg a day to accommodate their lower oestrogen levels and decreased intestinal calcium absorption related to training (American Dietetic Association, 1987). Women who experience a heavy menstrual flow may have increased requirements for iron and the vitamins associated with blood formation.

While there is some evidence to suggest that exercise increases requirements for certain vitamins and minerals (for example chromium) involved in energy metabolism and oxidation, it is generally agreed that the vitamin and mineral needs of most athletes can be met from a varied diet. Indiscriminate supplementation can lead to nutritional imbalances. Where there is doubt about the nutritional adequacy of a diet, a basic multi-vitamin, multi-mineral supplement could be advised.

Fluid

Fluid losses during exercises are inevitable but losses of more than 2% of body weight have been shown to affect athletic performance. To minimize dehydration, the body should be fully hydrated before taking exercise. An effort should be made to drink small amounts of fluids at regular intervals during exercise and then to drink plenty of fluid as soon as possible after exercise. Those taking exercise should not wait until they feel thirsty before they drink.

The amount of electrolytes lost in sweat is very small and there is little evidence that they need to be replaced during exercise by electrolyte drinks. Whilst small amounts of salt or glucose may help to increase the rate of fluid absorption, there is seldom a good enough reason to use these drinks in place of plain water.

Water is ideal; alternatively very dilute fruit juice or fruit squash can be drunk. A high osmolar drink (greater than 5% osmolarity) will reduce the rate of fluid absorption, as will large volumes of liquid. Colder drinks (5°C) tend to be absorbed more rapidly.

Salt tablets should be avoided and there is ample salt present naturally in foods without having to take extra salt at mealtimes (Wootton, 1988).

Ergogenic aids

There is an enormous range of nutritional substances used as ergogenic aids in sport. Some may have no proven value or even any scientific basis for their claimed effectiveness. Popular aids include ginseng, bee pollen, brewer's yeast, wheatgerm, lecithin, honey, amino acid supplements and kelp. If individuals are determined to continue taking such foods or supplements it is important to ensure that they also continue to follow a sound nutritional eating pattern.

Ergogenic aids, despite their impressive-sounding claims, are no substitute for a healthy balanced diet, hard and consistent training, and adequate rest (Bean, 1993). Undesirable side-effects may exist and the long-term effects of such supplements on health have not been fully tested.

The role of primary health care

Although the majority of the population would benefit from more exercise, a small proportion of the population exercise regularly and may seek advice from the practice team on various aspects of their diet and health in the context of their chosen sport.

General advice on diet

The most suitable diet for those who are physically active is that recommended for the general population, namely a diet containing plenty of starchy high fibre foods, fruit and vegetables, together with moderate amounts of milk, milk products and meat or alternatives such as poultry, fish, pulses and nuts (see Appendix 1 and Part 1, page 31).

Female athletes

Female athletes generally require less energy than males, but require more iron (Wootton, 1988; Bean, 1993). With regard to energy needs, not only are women smaller, but relatively less of their body mass is lean tissue. Low iron intakes can be associated with low energy intakes. The latter are particularly common among women athletes whose sport requires a relatively low body weight, for example middle and long distance runners, ballet dancers and gymnasts, who may voluntarily restrict their food intake. Low iron intakes are also sometimes seen in vegetarians.

Poor iron intake results in iron deficiency anaemia, early symptoms of which (fatigue, headaches and impaired performance) often go unnoticed. Consequently, advice should be given to all women engaged in sports about the need for regular intakes of iron-rich food (see pages 34 and 78 and Part 1, page 29, for sources of iron).

Menstrual irregularities

The restricted diet of some female athletes may also be a contributing factor in the development of menstrual irregularities, and women who exercise intensively and regularly often show such irregularities and, sometimes, prolonged amenorrhoea. Wootton (1988) suggests that 50% of competitive female endurance runners and 44% of professional ballet dancers suffer profound disturbances in their menstrual cycles. On the other hand, sports where body weight is less important are associated with lower incidences: for example 12% of swimmers and cyclists.

The underlying cause of this disturbance is unclear, but is thought to involve interaction between exercise, body weight and diet.

Menstrual irregularities can also have adverse effects on bone density (see Chapter 11) since circulating oestrogen levels are low (oestrogen promotes calcification of bones). In such women, it is important that an adequate intake of calcium is maintained. The reference nutrient intake for teenage girls up to the age of 18 is 800 mg daily (see Part 1, Appendix 2).

Young athletes

One means of encouraging adolescents to improve their diets, which are frequently unbalanced with respect to fat, sugar and fibre, is to link the need for good nutrition with physical activity.

Eating disorders are often observed in young female athletes such as gymnasts and ballet dancers attempting to control their weight (see page 55 and Part 3, Eating Disorders). What starts out as simple calorie counting may easily get out of hand and can unfortunately be missed by coaches and parents alike.

The temperature-regulating capacity of pre-pubescent athletes when exercising in the heat is considerably less than that of adults because sweat glands in the skin are not fully developed. Therefore young athletes are more prone to heat exhaustion (Wootton, 1988) and the need for plenty of fluid should be stressed.

Vegetarian diets

The popularity of vegetarianism has increased dramatically in recent years, particularly among the athletic community. Potential deficiencies can be prevented by ensuring that sufficient alternative sources of iron are eaten (for example green leafy vegetables, wholegrain cereals, beans and nuts). Consumption of foods rich in vitamin C will improve the absorption of iron from cereal and vegetable foods eaten at the same meal. Vegans usually need to take B_{12} supplements (see Chapter 7).

Although a vegetarian diet can be a perfectly healthy way of eating, it is not necessary to be vegetarian in order to improve athletic performance.

Books by Wootton (1988) and Bean (1993) and an information sheet by the British Dietetic Association (1990) offer more detailed responses to some of the questions which primary health care professionals may be asked.

References

American Dietetic Association (1987) Nutrition for physical fitness — a statement by ADA. *Journal of the American Dietetic Association* **76,** 437–43.

Bean A (1993) *The Complete Guide to Sports Nutrition*. London, A and C Black.

British Dietetic Association, Community Nutrition Group (1990) *Nutrition and Sport Performance. Information Sheet No. 18*. Birmingham, BDA.

Department of Health, Committee on the Medical Aspects of Food Policy (1991) *Dietary Reference Values for Food Energy and Nutrients for the United Kingdom. Report on Health and Social Subjects 41*. London, HMSO.

Wootton S (1988) *Nutrition for Sport*. London, Simon and Schuster.

Section 3:
The Prevention of Ill Health

10

Coronary heart disease

Key points

1. Rates of coronary heart disease (CHD) began to fall gradually in the 1970s, but the disease remains the major cause of death in men and the second major cause of death in women today. The UK as a whole is near the top of the international league table for coronary heart disease. Northern Ireland and Scotland are at the top.

2. The *Health of the Nation* document has identified poor diet as a major and modifiable influence on the principal risk factors for coronary heart disease. Improvements in diet are therefore central to prevention. The disease processes involved in coronary heart disease are multifactorial, so several other causes must also be tackled in prevention strategies, for example smoking and physical inactivity. Several risk factors, which may not be causal but indicative of likely disease, are recognized, for example family history, age, and sex.

3. The four principal modifiable factors leading to coronary heart disease are smoking, hypertension, a high plasma level of low density lipoprotein cholesterol and physical inactivity. These interact synergistically in Britain to increase the risk of coronary heart disease markedly: studies in Japan and China show that severe hypertension and smoking have a limited capacity to induce coronary heart disease unless dietary factors, which induce a rise in cholesterol levels, are also present; the lower the blood cholesterol, the lower the risk of coronary heart disease. The atherosclerosis which underlies coronary heart disease develops over decades but short-term effects relate to thrombosis. Thus

benefits of behavioural change are evident within months and major benefit is seen within five years, mainly through effects on thrombosis and limiting the progression of atherosclerosis.

4. Only 11%–12% of British adults are free from all the principal risk factors: smoking, hypertension, hypercholesterolaemia and inactivity. Over three-quarters of middle-aged adults in Britain have cholesterol levels >5.2 mmol/l, which is the upper limit for an acceptable level; currently 23% of all British adults have substantial hypercholesterolaemia, that is cholesterol >6.8 mmol/l; a national strategy to improve the quality of the diet should involve everybody. In addition, those with one of these three principal risk factors should be identified and receive special advice. If the average intake of saturates in Britain fell from 16% to the recommended 11%, the expressed prevalence of marked hypercholesterolaemia would be expected to fall from 23% to 6%.

5. The three classic risk factors, smoking, hypertension and hypercholesterolaemia, together account for half the variation in CHD rates. The other half remains unexplained but may relate to the impact of antioxidants, for example vitamins E and C derived from vegetables, fruits and vegetable oils, on blood clotting and the processes leading to atherosclerosis and the impact of physical inactivity.

6. Saturates from C_{12} to C_{16} chain lengths have been directly linked to the elevation in LDL cholesterol, although the evidence for C_{12} is less clear. Polyunsaturates (PUFA) of the n-6 series lower LDL cholesterol. Dietary cholesterol is less important than dietary

saturates but trans fatty acids, for example, derived from chemically hardened fats, can raise LDL cholesterol as well as having other adverse effects, for example on PUFA metabolism, and other lipoproteins, such as Lp(a), which are linked to thrombosis. Long chain n-3 fatty acids lower plasma triglycerides and have potential anti-thrombotic and anti-arrhythmia effects.

7. Genetic factors contribute to CHD risk and mostly explain the familial aggregation of coronary heart disease. The genetic factors often modify the sensitivity to important dietary factors; thus only in rare (<1 in 500) individuals with familial hypercholesterolaemia does diet prove relatively ineffective.

8. There is good evidence that dietary sodium (mostly as salt) is important in determining levels of blood pressure and in particular the rise in blood pressure with age. Blood pressure is also increased by alcohol, by low potassium intakes, by modest increases in weight and particularly by abdominal obesity. Thus, modest weight reduction, for example 5–10 kg, and particularly in those with abdominal obesity, can have a substantial impact on hypertension. Increasing the dietary polyunsaturates to saturates ratio also reduces blood pressure.

9. A high total fat intake increases the risk of obesity, and therefore of hypertension and diabetes, both of which are strong promoters of coronary heart disease. These links explain the renewed emphasis on reducing total fat intakes as well as modifying the types of fatty acid eaten.

10. Exercise is an important protective factor against coronary heart disease as well as against obesity, hypertension and non-insulin dependent diabetes mellitus. General activity, such as walking, is important; vigorous activity is best maintained throughout childhood and adult life and is particularly important in the elderly.

11. The latest Department of Health report on cardiovascular disease reiterates the importance of dietary change as a principal need for children (over age five years) and adults, and the need to stop smoking and to be more active (DH, 1994). European reports have the same advice which, on being implemented in Finland, reduced the number of people dependent on drugs to control hypertension by 75% and death rates from stroke fell by >60% over a 20-year period. CHD rates in men and women also fell to a similar extent, accompanied by a decline in plasma cholesterol and hypertension in both sexes and in smoking rates in men. The health gain to be expected from dietary change in a British practice is therefore considerable.

12. Patients with pre-existing coronary heart disease can halve their expected risk of subsequent coronary heart disease by dietary changes which increase their n-3 fatty acid intake; the risk of cardiac arrhythmia is particularly reduced. Cholesterol screening is not necessary as a routine procedure but should be used in the screening of relatives of those who develop premature coronary heart disease.

The size of the problem

Coronary heart disease still heads the list of causes of death in men (30%), resulting in more deaths than cancer (27%) and stroke. It is the second major cause of death, after cancer, in women. This is in spite of deaths from coronary heart disease having gradually fallen in all age groups in men and women in England and Wales, Scotland and Northern Ireland since the 1970s (Gregory et al., 1990). In most age and sex categories, current mortality rates have been reduced to the levels seen in the 1950s, but death from coronary heart disease still remains the most common single cause of death during middle age in men.

Such is the concern about the significance of coronary heart disease as a cause of premature death in the UK, that the government has set Health of the Nations targets:

- To reduce the death rate for coronary heart disease in people under 65 by at least 40% by the year 2000 (from 58 per 100 000 population in 1990 to no more than 35 per 100 000)

- To reduce the death rate for coronary heart disease in people aged 65–74 by at least 30% by the year 2000 (from 899 per 100 000 population in 1990 to no more than 629 per 100 000).

To help achieve these aims, targets have been set for the reduction of the level of specific risk factors, for example blood pressure, obesity and smoking, and also for aspects of diet associated with these risk factors, for example fat and saturated fatty acid intake. These are described in more detail on page 102.

The extent of the problem should not be underestimated. The first in a series of government health surveys of adults in England (OPCS, 1993) indicated that only 12% of men and 11% of women are free from all of the four main risk factors (hypercholesterolaemia, high blood pressure, smoking and inactivity). About a third of both men and women have one risk factor; 36% of men and 34% of women have two risk factors; about 1 in 5 have high levels of three risk factors; and 2% of men (3% of women) have high levels of all four.

The proportion with three or more risk factors increases with age. Among men, it rises from 4% of 16–24 year olds to 44% of those over 75. In women, the corresponding figures are 6% and 61%. In both sexes, but particularly in women, there is a strong social class gradient in the chance of having three or four risk factors, the risk being lowest in social classes 1 and 2.

Differences in death rates within the UK

There are considerable variations in coronary mortality rates between UK regions, and between social classes and ethnic groups.

There is a north-west/south-east gradient in mortality rates. Not only are rates greater in Scotland and Northern Ireland, but within England death rates are also higher in the north than in the south. With the possible exception of smoking (see page 106), it has not been possible to correlate these geographical trends with the conventional major risk factors. Perhaps surprisingly, this gradient corresponds with a worldwide pattern in which CHD mortality rates increase with increasing distance from the equator (Fleck, 1989).

In the UK, and within this geographical gradient, urban areas tend to have much higher rates than rural areas. This is likely to be influenced by the independent trends seen with socio-economic groups: those in manual groups are more susceptible to coronary heart disease than those in non-manual occupations. In the British regional heart study, the rate of heart attacks (fatal and non-fatal) was 44% higher in a 6-year follow-up period in manual workers compared with non-manual workers (Pocock et al., 1987). Similarly, in the Whitehall study of civil servants, men in the lowest grade had three times the mortality of men in the highest grade over a 10-year period (Marmot et al., 1978). The study also found higher rates of smoking, more obesity, less leisure time physical activity, and higher blood pressure among the manual workers, and dietary differences such as lower vegetable and fruit consumption.

Bangladeshis, Gujaratis, Punjabis and South Indians living in London have mortality rates from coronary heart disease which are 40% higher than UK national average levels (McKeigue et al., 1991). This finding is not peculiar to people from the Indian subcontinent living in Britain; similar findings have been reported in South-East Asians living in many parts of the world. On the other hand, Afro-Caribbeans and people from sub-Saharan Africa have rates lower than the national UK average. These differences cannot be explained by differences in the classical risk factors for the disease (see page 111).

Table 10.1 *Health of the Nation targets for coronary heart disease*

Risk factor targets

- To reduce mean systolic blood pressure in the adult population by at least 5 mmHg by 2005

- To reduce the proportion of men and women aged 16–64 who are obese by at least 25% and 33% respectively by 2005

- To reduce the proportion of men drinking more than 21 units of alcohol per week and women drinking more than 14 units of alcohol per week by 30% by 2005

- To reduce the prevalence of cigarette smoking in men and women aged 16 and over to no more than 20% by the year 2000 (a reduction of at least 35% in men and 20% in women)

Nutrition targets

- To reduce the average percentage of food energy derived by the population from saturated fatty acids by at least 35% by 2005

- To reduce the average percentage of food energy derived from total fat by the population by at least 12% by 2005

Source: Department of Health (1992).

The range of risk factors

Coronary heart disease is clearly a multi-factorial disease which means that a number of characteristics can lead to its development (see page 103). There is still some debate as to the relative importance of the various identified risk factors. However, the government's Health of the Nation initiative has identified four major risk factors, each of which is capable of modification:

- smoking
- high blood cholesterol
- high blood pressure
- inactivity.

So far, targets have been set for two of these (Table 10.1). In addition, nutrition targets have been set for total fat intake and intake of saturates.

There is great confusion about the nature of the so-called 'risk factor'. The latest (1994)

Department of Health report notes that there are inherent biological traits, such as age, sex and family history, which indicate risk but cannot be changed (Table 10.2). Social characteristics, for example social class or ethnic group, are also markers of risk because of behavioural or other factors as well as for constitutional reasons. Behavioural factors, such as diet, smoking, alcoholic consumption and lack of physical activity, lead mechanistically to metabolic changes which are then causally related to the propensity to thrombosis and/or atherogenesis. Epidemiological studies repeatedly demonstrate throughout the world that those who smoke, have a raised blood pressure and elevated serum cholesterol levels show an increased likelihood of coronary heart disease. In China and Japan smoking and hypertension rates are high but CHD rates are very low: this is linked to their very low cholesterol levels – average total levels of 4 mmol/l with LDL cholesterol levels of 2 mmol/l compared with British levels of 6–7 mmol/l and 4–5 mmol/l respectively. In China cholesterol levels do not rise with age whereas in Britain the age effect is marked. However, even at the lower cholesterol levels seen in China there is a clear linear relationship between total blood cholesterol levels and the development of coronary heart disease.

The dietary approach to the prevention of heart disease has centred on the universally accepted link between intake of saturates, blood cholesterol (particularly LDL cholesterol) concentrations and coronary heart disease. This is sometimes referred to as the lipid hypothesis.

The 1994 COMA report on cardiovascular disease reiterates the conclusions of many earlier reports from the 1960s onwards. Only modest changes in the experts' conclusions have been made over several decades, for example a reduced emphasis on the need for high intakes of polyunsaturates, proposals to increase selectively consumption of n-3 polyunsaturates and a focus on trans fatty acids. Yet both the medical profession and the public are sometimes confused by articles putting undue emphasis on new findings or

Table 10.2 *Major risk factors for coronary heart disease*

Principal risk factors	Other risk factors
Modifiable: ★ Smoking ★ Hypertension (high blood pressure) ★ Hypercholesterolaemia (high blood cholesterol) ★ Insufficient exercise *Non-modifiable*: ★ Family history ★ Being male ★ Advancing age	★ Diabetes mellitus ★ Overweight and obesity (especially when fat accumulates around the internal organs) ★ Poor antioxidant intake ★ Haemostatic factors, e.g. high plasma fibrinogen ★ Psychosocial factors: socio-economic status, stress, personality type ★ Alcohol intake ★ Soft drinking water

Source: Buttriss et al. (1993).

particular points of view. Acknowledgement of the complex nature of the processes leading to coronary heart disease and the search for the unexplained part of the variation in the disease is often wrongly taken to indicate that the recognized risk factors no longer apply. Inevitably, in the search, conflicting evidence is reported. Disappointing as this process can be to those committed to prevention, such studies provide an opportunity to learn from past mistakes and to improve the impact of future interventions.

Table 10.3 summarizes a recent major re-analysis of the prospective studies and intervention trials which seek to assess the effects of reducing cholesterol levels in the blood.

A distinction must now clearly be made between drug trials and dietary intervention (Davey-Smith et al., 1993). Long-term studies on drugs usually reveal a marked fall in CHD rates but often only modest change in total mortality — because the drugs induce a variety of side-effects and other illnesses. Dietary intervention does not have these side-effects despite theories that it might. Thus, with dietary intervention there is no increase in cancer rates — the effect is one of delaying the incidence of CHD events from the ages of 40–60 until much later in life (Law et al., 1994a). The integrated data from many prospective studies (Table 10.3) imply that it is a mistake to ignore the benefit from changing the diet of those aged 60 or more. It

Table 10.3 *The predicted and observed fall in the incidence of or mortality from coronary heart disease with a 10% reduction in blood cholesterol levels*

Age (years)	Expected % reduction in risk of coronary heart disease		Observed fall in incidence (death or non-fatal infarct) after follow up for:		
	From long-term prospective studies	From international comparisons	2 years	2.1–5 years	>5 years
35–44	54	–			
45–54	39	–			
55–64	27	38	7	22	25
65–74	20	–			
75–84	19	–			

Source: Adapted from Law et al. (1994b).

is particularly beneficial to change the diet and activity patterns of retired men and women because the dietary changes can also be expected to reduce the chances of nutritional deficiencies, and help to avoid stroke, cataract and diabetes, as well as coronary heart disease.

Table 10.3 also includes information on the intervention trials which are usually conducted on middle-aged men. Improve-ments in risk are clear within 1–2 years, and after 5 years the net effect is almost as great as that experienced if the individual's cholesterol level had always been at the lower level.

The marked benefits of dietary change can also be seen from national statistics. Thus, in North-East Finland, unlike Britain, there has been a major campaign backed by the medi-cal profession and community workers to

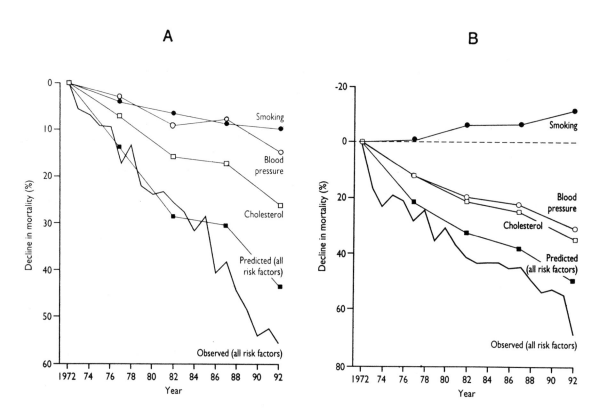

Changes in risk factors from 1972–1992

	Men		% of 1972 value	Women		% of 1972 value
	1972	1992		1972	1992	
Cholesterol mmol/l	6.78	5.90	(87)	6.72	5.54	(82)
Diastolic blood pressure (mmHg)	93	84	(90)	92	80	(87)
Proportion smokers %	53	37	(70)	11	20	(182)

Source: Vartiainen et al. (1994). Reproduced with permission of the BMJ Publishing Group.

Figure 10.1 *The predicted and observed death rates from coronary heart disease in (A) men and (B) women aged 35–64 in North-East Finland from 1972 to 1992*

change the diet by converting a very large proportion of the population from whole milk to semi-skimmed and skimmed milk, to introduce low fat spreads instead of butter and hard margarines, to reduce smoking and to more than double vegetable and fruit consumption. Fish intake has risen and a fall in salt consumption has also occurred. Whereas Table 10.3 relates only to hugely expensive and complex prospective and intervention trials conducted on men, it is now possible to look at data for both sexes in Eastern Karelia where risk factors and death rates were monitored over a 20-year period. Figures 10.1A and B show the precipitous fall in the observed CHD death rates and what would have been expected from the changes in smoking, high blood pressure rates and cholesterol levels. This fall in CHD rates is seen in women despite the recent worrying increase in smoking rates — a feature also seen in Britain. The data given in the notes below the figure show a fall in total cholesterol levels for the whole population which most doctors in Britain would consider impossible to achieve. Furthermore, the fall in blood pressure is remarkable. Other Finnish studies showed that blood pressure fell within a month of reducing the saturates and increasing the polyunsaturates content of the diet, the effect being especially marked in Finnish diets with polyunsaturates to saturates ratios of below 0.3 (Puska et al., 1985). Thus, not only have CHD rates fallen remarkably but in Finland there has also been a 75% reduction in those needing drug treatment for hypertension. The fall in stroke death rates in Finland of more than 60% over a 20-year period relates mainly to the fall in blood pressure (Vartiainen et al., 1995), whereas Figure 10.1 shows that cholesterol reduction has the greater effect on CHD rates. These remarkable changes do not, of course, mean that the effects relate solely to the fall in cholesterol, blood pressure and/or smoking. The dietary changes were many — in particular there has been a doubling in fruit, berry and vegetable consumption over the past two decades. But it does show that the current advice, based on concerns about cholesterol, blood pressure and smoking levels, can be highly effective.

Table 10.4 *Current nutrient intakes and average national UK targets proposed in 1994*

	Current average intake	Proposed average target
Total fat (%E)	41	35
Saturates	16	11
Polyunsaturates n-6 (%E)	6	No increase
n-3 (%E)	0.7	1.4
Trans fatty acids (%E)	2	<2
Monounsaturates (%E)	15	13
Dietary cholesterol (mg/day)	245	No increase
Carbohydrate (%E)	45	≈50
NSP (fibre) (g/day)	12	18
Salt (g/day)	9	6
Potassium (g/day)	2.5	3.5 (RNI)

Source: Based on DH (1994) and DH (1991).

From this one can conclude that there are opportunities for inducing a marked change in disease patterns in Britain and a primary health care team could expect to see a very considerable reduction in the burden of disease if prevention were to be made an important component of medical practice.

The latest COMA Report on Nutritional Aspects of Cardiovascular Disease (DH, 1994) sets a series of nutritional targets and also gives an example, in terms of national averages, of the extent of the changes needed to the national diet for these targets to be implemented. These changes do not apply to individuals, whose diets will inevitably be different from the 'national average' diet. Table 10.4 summarizes the nutritional targets, and practical dietary measures for individuals can be found in Part 1, page 33.

Practical management of CHD prevention

Practical ways of managing the prevention of coronary heart disease have recently been described in a consensus report by the European Societies of Cardiology, Atherosclerosis and Hypertension (Pyörälä et al.,

Table 10.5 *Priorities for coronary heart disease prevention in clinical practice*

1. Patients with established coronary heart disease or other atherosclerotic vascular disease

2. Asymptomatic patients with particularly high risk (those with severe hypercholesterolaemia or other form of dyslipidaemia, diabetes or hypertension, subjects with a cluster of several risk factors)

3. Close relatives of:
   - patients with early onset coronary heart disease or other atherosclerotic vascular disease
   - asymptomatic patients with particularly high risk

4. Other patients met in connection with ordinary clinical practice.

Source: Taken from Pyörälä et al. (1994).

1994). Table 10.5 sets out the sequence of priorities for CHD prevention in clinical practice. Clearly those who have established vascular disease need immediate secondary prevention. A familial history is also important and patients listed in Table 10.5 have a greater need for help than those picked up by routine or opportunistic screening. Figure 10.2 provides a simple way of predicting the chances of a man or women developing a coronary event, such as the onset of angina or having a myocardial infarct during a 10-year period. By selecting the sex and age and using three of the principal risk factors, it is possible to predict the risk of developing angina or having a myocardial infarct within the next 10-year period.

The scheme does not include a measure for physical activity although it has been shown repeatedly to protect against coronary heart disease even in those who smoke, are overweight or hypertensive or hypercholesterolaemic. The more exercise the less the risk, but an hour's brisk walking each day with about three 20-minute periods per week of more intensive exercise, such as bicycling, swimming or jogging, has a substantial benefit in reducing the risk of a myocardial infarct to a third of that seen in the completely inactive (Lakka et al., 1994).

Therefore the scheme set out in Figure 10.2, with some modification if the patient is particularly involved in sports or other heavy physical activity, can be used to provide a very clear perspective on the need for lifestyle changes. Some changes are comparatively simple and can be summarized as follows.

Smoking

A great effort is needed to help patients to give up smoking but dietary advice is required whether or not they succeed because British smokers have a particularly bad diet and some of the abnormalities induced by smoking can be reversed by a suitable change in nutrient intake. Those giving up smoking will usually need dietary advice anyway because the common weight gain after stopping smoking needs to be combated by a diet low in fat and sugar and rich in vegetables, fruit and wholegrain cereals. One reason for women persisting with smoking is their fear of weight gain if they stop smoking — smoking not only suppresses appetite but increases the metabolic rate.

Hypertension

Moderate hypertension can often be treated by lifestyle changes alone: a modest 5-10 kg weight loss, even in those at the upper end of the 'normal' range of body mass index (BMI) 20–25, can have a marked effect, particularly if there is abdominal obesity. A systematic reduction in salt intake – not simply by reducing salt use at table or in the kitchen (which amounts to only 15% of intake), but by a careful avoidance of high salt foods, for example some cereals such as All-bran, extracts such as Marmite, and smoked/salted foods, for example bacon, prepared meats, pies, crisps and many biscuits. Blood pressure falls in proportion to the magnitude of the reduction and takes time (Law et al., 1991). A reduction in fat, particularly saturates, also has an effect. If these dietary changes are combined with regular exercise, the fall in blood pressure can reduce the need for hypertensive drugs by 60% over the following decade (Stamler et al., 1980).

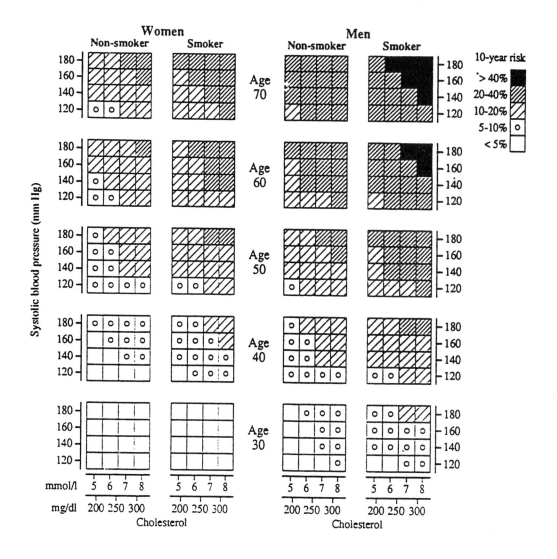

- To find a person's absolute 10-year risk of a CHD event, find the table for sex, age and smoking status. Inside the table, find the cell nearest to the person's systolic blood pressure (mmHg) and cholesterol (mmol/l or mg/dl).

- To find a person's relative risk, compare the risk category with other people of the same age. The absolute risk shown here may not apply to all populations, especially those with a low CHD incidence. Relative risk is likely to apply to most populations.

- The effect of changing cholesterol, smoking status or blood pressure can be read from the chart.

- The effect of lifetime exposure to risk factors can be seen by following the table upwards. This can be used when advising younger people.

- Risk is at least one category higher in people with overt cardiovascular disease. People with diabetes, familial hyperlipidaemia or a family history of premature cardiovascular disease are also at increased risk.

- Risks are shown for exact ages, blood pressures and cholesterols. Risk increases as a person approaches the next category.

- The tables assume HDL cholesterol to be 1.0 mmol/l in men (39 mg/dl) and 1.1 mmol/l (43 mg/dl) in women. People with lower levels of HDL cholesterol and/or with triglyceride levels above 2.3 mmol/l (200 mg/dl) are at higher risk.

- Cholesterol: 1 mmol/l=38.67 mg/dl.

Source: Pyörälä et al. (1994). Reproduced with permission of Elsevier Science Ltd, Ireland.

Figure 10.2 *Coronary risk chart based on a risk function derived from the Framingham Study (Anderson et al., 1991)*

Table 10.6 Lipid-lowering diet (adapted from the European Atherosclerosis Society recommendations, 1992)

	Recommended foods*	Foods for use in moderation†	Foods to be avoided‡
Cereals	Wholegrain bread, wholegrain breakfast cereals, porridge, cereals, pasta, crispbread, matzo, rice		Croissant, brioche
Dairy products	Skimmed milk, very low-fat cheeses, e.g. cottage cheese, fat-free fromage frais or quark, very low-fat yogurt	Semi-skimmed milk, low-fat yogurt, fat-reduced and lower fat cheeses, e.g. Brie, Camembert, Edam, reduced fat Cheddar, Gouda, feta, ricotta,	Whole milk, condensed milk, cream, imitation milk, full-fat cheeses, full-fat yogurt
Eggs	Egg white, egg substitutes	Two whole eggs per week	
Soups	Consommés, vegetable soups		Thickened soups, cream soups
Fish	All white and oily fish (grilled, poached, smoked). Avoid skin (e.g. on sardines or whitebait)	Fish fried in suitable oils	Roe, fish fried in unknown or unsuitable oils or fats
Shellfish	Oysters, scallops	Mussels, lobster, scampi	Prawns, shrimps, calamari
Meat	Turkey, chicken (avoid skin), veal, game, rabbit, spring lamb, very lean beef. Do not use fat in cooking	Lean beef, ham, bacon, lamb (once or twice a week). Veal or chicken sausage. Liver twice a month	Duck, goose, all visibly fatty meats, usual sausages, salamis, meat pies, pâtés, poultry skin
Fats		Polyunsaturated oils, e.g. sunflower, corn, walnut, safflower Mono-unsaturated oils (olive oil, rape-seed oil). Soft (unhydrogenated) margarines based on permitted oils, especially low fat spreads	Butter, suet, lard, dripping, palm oil, hard margarines, hydrogenated fats
Vegetables and fruit	All fresh and frozen vegetables, emphasis on legumes: beans, lentils, chick peas, sweetcorn, boiled or jacket potatoes, all fresh or dried fruit, tinned fruit (unsweetened)	Roast or chipped potatoes cooked in permitted oils	Roast or chipped potatoes, vegetables or rice fried in unknown or unsuitable oils or fats, potato crisps, oven chips, salted tinned vegetables
Desserts	Sorbet, jellies, puddings based on skimmed milk, fruit salads, meringue		Ice cream, puddings, dumplings, sauces based on cream or butter
Baked foods		Pastry, biscuits prepared with unsaturated margarine or oils	Commercial pastry, biscuits, commercial pies, snacks and puddings

Table 10.6 *continued*

Confectionery	Turkish delight, nougat, boiled sweets	Marzipan, halva	Chocolate, toffees, fudge, coconut bars, butterscotch
Nuts	Walnuts, almonds, chestnuts	Brazils, peanuts, pistachios	Cashews, coconut, salted nuts
Beverages	Tea, filter or instant coffee, water, calorie free soft drinks	Alcohol, low-fat chocolate drinks	Chocolate drinks, Irish coffee, full fat malted drinks, boiled coffee
Dressings, flavourings	Pepper, mustard herbs, spices	Low-fat salad dressings	Added salt, salad dressings, salad cream, mayonnaise

*Recommended foods are generally low in fat and/or high in fibre. These should be used regularly as part of the diet.

†Foods for use in moderation contain unsaturated fatty acids or smaller quantities of saturates. As the diet should be low in fat, these foods are allowed only in moderation.

‡Foods to be avoided contain large proportions of saturates and/or cholesterol, and therefore should be avoided wherever possible by those on a lipid-lowering diet for the treatment of hyperlipidaemia.

Source: Adapted from Pyörälä et al. (1994).

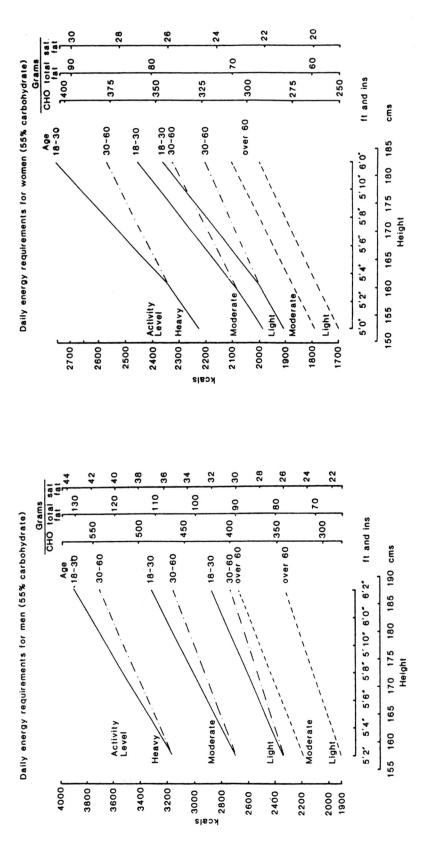

Figure 10.3

Source: Lean MJ and James WPT (1986) Prescription of diabetic diets in the 1980s. © The Lancet Ltd. Reproduced with permission. *Lancet* 1, 723–5.

Hyperlipidaemia

Table 10.6 is based on the practical guidelines from the European Atherosclerosis Society for the treatment of hyperlipidaemia. It has been known for decades that the higher the initial level of blood cholesterol the greater the response to a diet selectively low in saturates. A restriction of dietary cholesterol, for example from eggs and shellfish, is advocated for those with particularly high levels because mechanistically dietary cholesterol, although only moderately absorbed, seems to amplify the effects of saturates by restricting the liver clearance of LDL cholesterol. If blood triglycerides are elevated, alcohol intake will need particular restriction whilst exercise of moderate intensity and the consumption of n-3 fatty acids from fish are usually very effective in reducing the triglycerides to normal levels.

The dietary changes proposed will have other beneficial effects. The mechanisms underlying thrombosis are complex but it is generally agreed that a fall in total fat will limit the acute rise in the pro-clotting factor VII after a fatty meal; a fall in saturates, especially in the intake of stearic acid ($C_{18:0}$), for example found in beef fat, is also likely to be beneficial by reducing the tendency to thrombus formation. Avoiding hardened margarines and biscuits, pastries and pies made with oils and fats rich in trans fatty acids will reduce the levels of Lp(a) in the blood of those genetically programmed to synthesize this lipoprotein. High Lp(a) levels, measured by the latest techniques, predict a myocardial infarction in those with hypercholesterolaemia. Lp(a) is now known to limit the plasmin-induced clearance of clots and experimentally to promote the atherosclerotic process (DH, 1994).

An intake of n-3 fatty acids from fish also has a selective effect in limiting the chances of cardiac arrhythmia both experimentally and in post-infarction secondary prevention trials (see page 114). Oily fish, such as sardines, sprats, herring, mackerel, trout and salmon, should be particularly encouraged at least once a week, with fish being taken as a meal at least twice weekly.

The greater the dietary change, the greater the effects on blood lipids; the more marked the fall in the LDL/HDL cholesterol ratio, the slower the progression of atherosclerosis in clinical studies. With the most extreme dietary changes, for example with a contribution to energy intake from fat as low as 10%, as in parts of China, it is even possible to see the beginning of a slow reversal of the atherosclerotic process within a 2-year period.

Doctors should remember that the simple dispensing of a diet sheet is one of the least useful means of engaging patients in behavioural change. This is best undertaken by negotiated sequential small changes which can be incorporated into daily living. The use of standard 1000 kcal or 1200 kcal diets to assist weight loss is also unhelpful without a clear understanding of each patient's own calorie requirement. This cannot be predicted accurately but Figure 10.3 displays a crude graph for estimating energy needs. A diet which induces a 1000 kcal deficit is likely to lead to hunger and a metabolic drive to eat, whereas a 500 kcal deficit seems easier to sustain but can only lead to a 0.5 kg weight loss per week. A 10 kg weight loss leads to a permanent 300 kcal fall in energy requirements, so a sustained increase in exercise, for example an hour's brisk walking daily, would be needed to counteract this weight-relative fall in both basal metabolism and the lower cost of exercise.

Other factors affecting coronary heart disease

If the variation in coronary heart disease is related to cholesterol levels, blood pressure and smoking, then at least half the variability between groups can be explained. Much research is now concerned with attempts to unravel a number of epidemiological observations (see Buttriss et al., 1991 for a review). Some of these current discrepancies

Table 10.7 *Epidemiological observations that are not explained by 'the lipid hypothesis'*

- The greater risk of coronary heart disease in men than in women

- The enhanced risk of coronary heart disease in women after menopause

- The systematic fall in coronary heart disease rates in women in most countries despite a variety of changes in men's rates

- Social class differences

- Greater risk in the Asian population in the UK despite lower blood pressure, lower plasma cholesterol and less smoking

- The very low coronary heart disease rates in countries like France despite comparatively high saturated fatty acid intakes

- The progressive fall in coronary heart disease in the USA regardless of sex, race, region or work status

- The finding in cohort and case-control studies that fruit and vegetable or cereal consumption is protective with no link established for saturated fatty acid intake

- The lack of association between changes in P/S ratio (ratio of polyunsaturated fatty acids to saturated fatty acids) in the UK diet and changes in coronary heart disease mortality, and between P/S ratios in regions of the UK and coronary heart disease prevalence (for example, the relatively high P/S ratio and yet high incidence of coronary heart disease in Northern Ireland)

Source: Modified from James et al. (1989).

Table 10.8 *Some newer factors in the risk profile for coronary heart disease*

- Factors influencing blood haemostasis and thrombosis
  - blood fibrinogen
  - diet and thrombosis

- Lipid peroxidation and free radical damage
  - oxidized LDL and endothelial damage
  - protective role of antioxidant nutrients
  - iron as a pro-oxidant
  - plasma homocysteine levels: high levels may promote endothelial arterial damage. Folate may protect against this effect (Pancharuniti et al., 1994)

- Diet and cardiac arrhythmias

- Influence of maternal health

- Increased emphasis on factors associated with social status and stress

- Seasonal changes in plasma vitamin D_3 levels

Source: Buttriss et al. (1991).

are given in Table 10.7, and Table 10.8 lists some of the newer factors which are now being considered as possible explanations for some or all of the remaining half of the variability.

Dietary fats and cholesterol

As suggested by the report on dietary reference values, not all saturated fatty acids have an effect on serum cholesterol level (DH, 1991). Myristic acid containing 14 carbon atoms (C_{14}) has a major effect. Palmitic acid (C_{16}) has a lesser effect, and there is no evidence that saturated fatty acids of longer (stearic, C_{18}) or shorter (C_{10}, C_{12}) chain lengths have any effect (DH, 1991). However, stearic acid is thought to promote blood clotting (see page 111). The main sources of C_{14} and C_{16} are chiefly animal fats such as milk fat, butter, meat fat, meat products. But coconut oil is also a rich source, as are many margarines and baked cereal products.

The n-6 or omega-6 family of polyunsaturates (linoleic acid and its derivatives) lower plasma cholesterol (both LDL and total cholesterol). The n-3 or omega-3 family (linolenic acid and its derivatives) have no effect on plasma cholesterol, but may inhibit clot formation.

Both n-6 polyunsaturates (for example as found in sunflower and corn oils and some soft margarines) and the n-3 polyunsaturates commonly found in oily fish appear capable of reducing the vulnerability of the heart to fibrillation during a period of ischaemia — a cause of sudden death. Long chain n-3 fatty acids appear particularly potent and Charnock (1994) suggests that the greatest benefit might be expected in populations regularly consuming fish (see page 114 regarding fatty fish and secondary prevention).

Intakes of polyunsaturates over 10% of dietary energy, by individuals, are not advisable (DH, 1991). The average intake of polyunsaturates has been set at the current average intake (6% of dietary energy), suggesting that no further increase in polyunsaturates is warranted. Polyunsaturates are vulnerable to peroxidation and concern has been expressed that a high intake of polyunsaturates coupled with inadequate protection by dietary antioxidant, such as vitamins E and C, may predispose to tissue damage (see pages 118–120). Although mechanisms have been proposed to explain how lipid peroxidation might result in coronary heart disease, as yet there is no direct evidence that high intakes of polyunsaturates provoke disease.

Dietary cholesterol has only a small effect on blood cholesterol levels, except in those few individuals with familial hypercholesterolaemia.

The Dietary Reference Values Report has concluded that there is insufficient evidence that a specific increase in the intake of monounsaturated fatty acids would help to prevent coronary heart disease (DH, 1991). Nevertheless, some studies have shown them to be as effective in lowering cholesterol levels as polyunsaturates, such as linoleic acid (Jackson et al., 1984; Kohlmeier et al., 1985; Kwiterovitch et al., 1985; Mattson and Grundy, 1985). Unlike polyunsaturates (at high intakes), monounsaturates have the additional advantage of not lowering blood levels of 'protective' HDL cholesterol and are not as susceptible as polyunsaturates to oxidation (see page 118). Oleic acid, the major monounsaturate in the diet, is found in large amounts in olive oil and other vegetable oils such as rape-seed oil. It is also present in meat and milk fat.

For some time it has been thought that the body metabolizes the trans isomers of unsaturated fatty acids in a way similar to that used with saturates (BNF, 1987). New research derived from the well-known Harvard Nurses Health Study has indicated that high intakes of trans fatty acids (particularly those formed when vegetable oils are hardened — hydrogenated) may promote the development of coronary heart disease (Willett et al., 1993). In this prospective study, women with the highest intakes of trans fatty acids of this type had the highest incidence of heart disease over the next eight years. Ascherio et al. (1994) have observed a highly significant association in both men and women between trans fatty acid intake and myocardial infarction even after adjusting for established coronary risk factors. Intake of margarine was again directly associated in this study.

A previous study among men had looked at the effect of trans fatty acids on blood cholesterol levels, finding an increase in the ratio of LDL cholesterol to HDL cholesterol which they predicted would correspond with a 27% increase in heart attack risk (Troisi et al., 1992). Mensink and Katan (1990) have reported similar findings, and evidence is accumulating that dietary trans fatty acids are able to increase plasma levels of lipoprotein (a) (Lp(a)), which is regarded as an independent risk factor for coronary heart disease. High concentrations of this lipoprotein are thought to increase both thrombogenesis and atherosclerosis (Mensink et al., 1992; Nestel et al., 1992), and Wahle and James (1993) have suggested that hydrogenated oils may predispose to thrombogenesis.

Intakes of trans fatty acids vary, and this is related to the lifestyle and socio-economic factors which influence food choice. The trans content of the cheaper margarines is quite high and so people who consume these in quantity and also eat lots of processed foods and fried take-away meals are likely to have higher intakes of this type of fatty acid. Willett's study showed that women who eat a lot of foods containing trans fatty acids have a 50% greater risk of heart disease than those who eat few. The profile of trans fatty acids found naturally in meat and milk fat is different and they are present in smaller amounts; and there was no relationship between their intake and risk of coronary heart disease.

Although recent evidence suggests that trans fatty acids may have a detrimental effect on human health and possibly on human growth and development, the findings are not yet absolutely definite (Wahle, 1994). Nevertheless, it would seem prudent to advise reduction in the consumption of trans fatty acids, particularly those in hydrogenated oils and their products. (For more information on dietary fat intake, see Part 1, pages 11–13.)

Fatty fish

Fish oils derived from fatty fish are rich in the n-3 polyunsaturates, eicosapentaenoic acid (EPA) and docosahexaenoic acid (DHA). These reduce plasma triglyceride concentrations. Results from the Diet and Re-infarction Trial (DART) indicated that fatty fish, eaten at least twice a week, resulted in fewer deaths among middle-aged men who had already had a heart attack than did either a low fat regimen (30% energy from fat, P/S ratio 1.0) or a high fibre regimen (cereal fibre intake doubled to 18 g/day) (Burr et al., 1989). This effect was seen after only 6 months and mortality was 29% lower after 2 years on the diet, which is suggestive of an effect on blood clotting rather than reduction in atherosclerosis. However, the precise mechanism by which fatty fish influences thrombosis is still unclear. It has been suggested that the effect may actually be on 'sudden death' and not infarction (MRC, 1991) (see page 111).

Researchers in Denmark have shown an association between high adipose tissue levels of DHA and low levels of coronary artery disease (Seidelin et al., 1992). The fatty acid composition of adipose tissue is thought to reflect the long-term fatty acid composition of the diet.

Soluble fibre

Despite the accumulating evidence to suggest that oats and other sources of soluble fibre

(a form of non-starch polysaccharide, NSP), such as guar gum, rye, barley and pulses, can reduce plasma cholesterol, the mechanism of the response remains unclear. Various suggestions have been made: soluble fibre may bind to cholesterol and bile acids, preventing their reabsorption and so the amount of cholesterol in circulation; soluble fibre is subject to bacterial fermentation in the colon, during which propionic acid, a short chain fatty acid capable of inhibiting cholesterol synthesis in the liver, is formed; soluble fibre slows glucose absorption and hence insulin release, which might reduce cholesterol synthesis. (For a review, see BNF, 1990.)

Coffee

The hazard of coffee drinking in relation to coronary heart disease has been speculated on for some years, but research findings have been inconsistent. A recent large prospective study of 45 000 men found no relationship between coffee consumption and either myocardial infarction or risk of stroke (Grobee et al., 1990). Overall, coffee does not seem to be a significant risk factor except in some Scandinavian countries where the use of unfiltered coffee leads to higher cholesterol levels.

Antioxidant nutrients and free radical damage

Attention is also now focusing on the role of free radical damage in coronary heart disease and the importance of dietary antioxidant status in preventing this damage (see page 118).

The body has evolved a complex interrelated protective system to prevent oxidative damage caused by free radical attack (see Buttriss et al., 1991). The system is centred around certain micronutrients which are often termed the antioxidant nutrients. These include certain metals (copper, zinc, manganese and selenium) which act as co-factors for antioxidant enzymes, and vitamins (vitamins C and E, beta-carotene) with specific antioxidant functions (see Table 10.9). (See also pages 118–120.)

Table 10.9 *The 'antioxidant nutrients' involved in protection against oxygen-free radicals – function and food sources*

Minerals	Function	Food sources
Copper	Component of superoxide dismutase* in cell cytoplasm. Also a component of caeruloplasmin, which converts ferrous iron to ferric iron. (It is ferrous iron which catalyzes free radical reactions)	Wholegrain cereals, meat, vegetables
Zinc	Component of superoxide dismutase* in cell cytoplasm	Meat, milk, cheese, bread, cereal products
Manganese	Component of superoxide dismutase* in cell mitochondrion	Wholegrain cereals and bread, nuts, vegetables, teas
Selenium	Component of glutathione peroxidation	Cereals, especially bread; fish, liver, pork, cheese, eggs, walnuts and brazil nuts
Vitamins		
E (specifically alpha-tocopherol)	Interferes with the lipid peroxidation chain reaction by combining with the oxygen free radical, preventing it from combining with the next fatty acid in the chain	Oil, particularly sunflower seed oil, almonds and hazel nuts, wholegrain breakfast cereals, wholegrain bread, dark green vegetables, eggs, margarine, cheese and dairy products
C	Scavenges free radicals Regenerates alpha-tocopherol	Fruit and vegetables, particularly kiwi fruit, black-currants, strawberries, green peppers, bean sprouts, new potatoes
Beta-carotene and other carotenoids	Scavenge free radicals	Yellow and orange fruit, green vegetables, e.g. carrots, apricots and pumpkins, spinach watercress, whole milk and its products
A	Scavenges singlet oxygen	Liver, whole milk and its products, butter, fortified margarine

*Enzyme which removes 'superoxide' but generates hydrogen peroxide.

Source: Buttriss et al. (1991).

Dietary surveys in various countries have shown strong inverse correlations between mortality from coronary heart disease and intake of fresh fruit and vegetables and the intake of vitamins C, E and beta-carotene (Gey, 1986). In the WHO/MONICA project, which was designed to compare heart disease mortality in a number of countries, data have been collected on plasma antioxidant levels in middle-aged men from 16 European populations, in which the differences in age-specific mortality from coronary heart disease ranged six-fold. Two of the 'classical' risk factors, total plasma cholesterol and blood pressure, were found to be only weakly correlated with risk of coronary heart disease and surprisingly there was no significant correlation with smoking habit (Gey et al., 1991). The authors suggest that the latter finding might be explained by the fact that the known deleterious effects of smoking were balanced in Southern European populations by protective dietary factors such as vitamin E.

A strong inverse correlation was found between plasma vitamin E levels and coronary heart disease, and vitamin C showed a moderately strong inverse relationship. This is indicative of the function of vitamin E in protecting against lipid peroxide-induced endothelial damage and lipoprotein modification. Correlations were also found for vitamin A but were weaker, and the correlation was weak or absent for carotene and selenium (Gey et al., 1991). However, recent work (Salonen et al., 1991; Suadicani et al., 1992) has indicated that selenium might be important after all in reducing heart disease risk, in at least some circumstances.

In two major prospective studies, one in men (Rimm et al., 1993) and the other in women (Stampfer et al., 1993), high intakes of vitamin E were associated with a reduced incidence of coronary heart disease; but further research is needed before supplements should be advised. New international analyses also suggest that vitamin E may explain the so-called French paradox of very low CHD rates despite appreciable intakes of saturates (see below).

Alcohol intake

A number of studies have shown an apparent protective association between light to moderate alcohol consumption and coronary heart disease. Shaper et al. (1988) argue that abstainers from alcohol are often ex-drinkers who tend to have more ill health. In a case-control population based study, Jackson et al.

(1991) showed that there was no evidence that the protective association was due to migration of former drinkers to non-drinking groups.

People who drink moderate amounts of alcohol have lower fibrinogen levels (although it has not been shown that alcohol reduces fibrinogen), and alcohol intake is associated with a decreased tendency of platelets to aggregate (Renaud et al., 1992). Hence, moderate amounts of alcohol may reduce thrombogenesis. Alcohol in moderation is also associated with raised HDL cholesterol levels.

Renaud and De Lorgeril (1992) have proposed that alcohol may explain the French paradox of low coronary death rates in spite of relatively high risk factor levels. It has also been proposed that phenolic compounds (flavonoids) in red wine, which have antioxidant properties, may also have beneficial effects on coronary risk (Frankel et al., 1993) by combating oxidation of LDL (see pages 118–120). Bellizzi et al. (1994), however, suggest that alcohol is not the principal factor — wine is better related to low CHD rates than alcohol *per se*, but longitudinal analyses suggest that the alpha-tocopherol component of vitamin E is the better predictor. Sources are shown in Table 10.9. A similar relationship is seen in Switzerland.

Alcohol abuse is a major cause of premature death and it is not possible to predict which individuals will progress from moderate use of alcoholic drinks to abuse. Thus, recommendations to the general public to increase their alcohol intake are not warranted (see Part 1, page 8).

Obesity and overweight

Although obesity is often not considered as an independent risk factor for coronary heart disease it does lead to the increase in blood pressure, serum cholesterol and diabetes which is crucially important in determining disease, so excess weight should be avoided (Manson, 1990; see Chapter 12). The selective accumulation of fat within the abdomen is, however, an even more important risk. Fat distribution around the waist rather than the hips, more than excess body weight alone, predicts a variety of metabolic problems, including diabetes, coronary heart disease, breast cancer and gall bladder disease (Ashwell, 1991).

Differences in fat distribution have been suggested as the main explanation of the differences seen in coronary mortality rates between men and women (Larsson et al., 1992). Centrally distributed fat is not necessarily a causal factor; it may merely be a marker for some other factor. However, it has been suggested that excess quantities of fatty acids from the abdominal fat travel directly via the portal vein to the liver and subsequently interfere with liver metabolism.

Overweight and obesity have been increasing rapidly in recent years. In 1993 over half the adults in England were overweight or obese — 57% of men and 48% of women (Bennett et al., 1995). Although a greater proportion of men are overweight (BMI over 25), women are more likely to be obese (BMI over 30) — 13% of men and 16% of women are now classed as obese. An earlier survey in 1986/87 had shown that 8% of men and 13% of women (aged 16–64) were obese. This dramatic increase over such a short period will make the Health of the Nation target for obesity even more difficult to achieve.

Among both men and women, body mass index is significantly associated with age, social class, and educational qualification level. The proportion of men and women with a body mass index of more than 25 peaks at age 45–64 for men (67%–70%) and 55–74 for women (59%–60%), and then decreases among older age groups. The proportion considered obese is highest in the 45–64 age groups (OPCS, 1993). Both body mass index and waist to hip ratio (a measure of centrally distributed fat) are higher in men and women with no educational qualifications.

Physical inactivity

Although physical activity does not appear to alter levels of blood total cholesterol to any great extent, it does have a beneficial effect on increasing HDL cholesterol which is suggested to protect against coronary heart disease (Hardman et al., 1989). Cardiovascular fitness, skeletal muscle strength and general well-being are also improved. The Health Education Authority (1990) recommends three 20-minute bouts of vigorous exercise per week. This exercise should be sufficient to raise the pulse rate and produce moderate breathlessness.

However, a recent survey (HEA, 1992) indicates that although 80% of the adult population believe themselves to be fit:

- a third of men and two-thirds of women find walking at a reasonable pace up a 1:20 slope physically demanding and a cause of breathlessness

- sustaining a reasonable pace for several minutes on level ground constitutes severe exertion for 50% of women over 55 years

- 30% of men and 50% of women aged 65–74 years have insufficient strength in their thigh muscles to rise from a chair without using their arms

- 40% of 65–74 year olds are inactive compared to less than 10% of 16–24 year olds

- the physical activity level of 70% of men and 91% of women aged 16–24 years is below that necessary for a fit and active life.

Fibrinogen and blood haemostasis

Recent research suggests that the role of other risk factors, such as those affecting blood haemostasis, should be given more attention. Many of the factors which are generally accepted as being predictive of coronary heart disease are also associated with an increase in fibrinogen levels (Ernst, 1990). These include smoking, high blood pressure, elevated plasma cholesterol, age, diabetes, obesity (increasing body mass index), male gender, oral contraceptives, low socio-economic status and possibly stress. Ernst suggests that fibrinogen is at least as predictive of coronary disease as plasma cholesterol.

Maternal and infant nutrition

Barker (1992) has proposed that cardio-vascular disease may have its origins in adverse conditions in early childhood. He and colleagues have linked the ratio of birth-weight to placental weight with risk of sub-sequent hypertension in adulthood (Barker et al., 1990) — higher birthweight/lower placental weight reduced the risk. They have also shown that incidence of adult onset diabetes can be predicted by low birthweight and poor growth during infancy (Hales et al., 1991), as can high fibrinogen levels, and nutrition in the first year of life can influence blood cholesterol (Fall et al., 1992).

Similarly, predictive of cardiovascular disease are a small head circumference, thinness at birth (Barker et al., 1993a) and a small ab-dominal girth (Barker et al., 1993b). It is suggested that these each reflect poor fetal growth. Associated with this are changes or poor development in certain tissues, includ-ing blood vessels, the pancreas and the liver. It is speculated that these changes pro-gramme glucose and insulin metabolism, blood pressure and LDL cholesterol concen-trations, and through these influence the risk of cardiovascular disease in later life.

The extensive body of evidence now pub-lished by this group of researchers serves to underline the importance of good nutrition prior to conception, during pregnancy and breast feeding, and during early infancy, and the impact poor nutrition during these critical periods may have on the health of the offspring during adulthood.

Associated pathological changes

The pathological changes associated with the development of coronary heart disease take place over many years. In simple terms, these changes can be considered to be: initial arterial injury, development of a fibrous plaque at the site of injury, blood clot forma-tion and the heart attack itself. These changes arise from a series of abnormal physiological responses which are influenced by a wide array of factors — some genetic, some age-related, some lifestyle-related, and some associated with diet. The incidence of coronary heart disease cannot therefore be attributed to any single aspect, let alone a component of diet.

The abnormal physiological conditions which affect the frequency and severity of injury to the coronary arteries include increased blood pressure, increased lipid oxidation (see page 114), an increased tendency for platelets to aggregate and an increased inflammatory res-ponse (see BNF, 1993). In turn, these are influenced by components of diet. For example, blood pressure is increased by high salt intake, the ratio of sodium to potassium intake, alcohol intake and obesity. Lipid oxidation is affected by the oxidizability of the fatty acids in low density lipoprotein particles (polyunsaturates are most prone to oxidation) and the balance between pro-oxidants (for example free copper and iron) and antioxidants (for example vitamins E and C and beta-carotene). The tendency for platelets to aggregate and for inflammation to occur are reduced by increased intake of the type of fatty acid found in oily fish, such as mackerel (see page 111).

The build up of the fibrous plaque in the injured artery wall is determined by a series of factors which affect both lipid and throm-bus deposition, for example raised plasma cholesterol (influenced by the fat, fatty acid and soluble fibre content of the diet), increased plasma fibrinogen (probably not affected by diet, though influenced by smoking), and increased plasma insulin levels (associated with centrally located fat deposition).

The formation of a major thrombus and the severity of the heart attack will be influenced by factors which affect blood coagulation and the regularity of the heart beat.

A concept that is gaining considerable support, sometimes referred to as the 'anti-oxidant hypothesis' or 'oxidized LDL

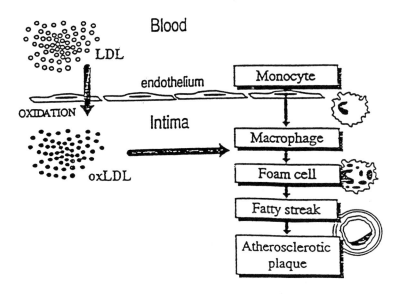

Figure 10.4 *The oxidized LDL hypotheses*

Source: Brown (1992). Reproduced with permission.

hypothesis', helps draw together some of these strands and suggests a mechanism by which atherosclerosis progresses and perhaps even how the initial injury to the artery occurs (Figure 10.4).

Although high levels of cholesterol-rich low density lipoprotein (LDL) particles in the plasma are strongly associated with an increased risk of coronary heart disease, these particles are not atherogenic in themselves (Brown, 1992). Although they can enter the blood vessel wall, they do not create an inflammatory reaction or tissue damage. By contrast, LDL particles which have been modified by oxidation are no longer recognized by the LDL receptors on the cell surface and behave akin to foreign material, in that they provoke an inflammatory response and so are ingested by macrophages as a means of removing them from the system. Once ingested they are cytotoxic and the macrophage is converted eventually into a foam cell, characteristic of fatty streaks, an early sign of damage to the artery wall.

There is evidence that these fatty streaks can disappear again, but under appropriate con-

ditions may gradually develop into the raised atherosclerotic plaques characteristic of atherosclerosis. As damage progresses, ulceration can occur resulting in disruption of the endothelium, attracting platelets and other blood components which aggravate the damage. In addition, small pieces of tissue can become dislodged, thus forming the focus for development of a thrombus.

It is unclear how this oxidation comes about, but it is assumed that free radicals are involved. As part of normal metabolism, many cellular reactions produce highly reactive and potentially destructive free radicals, frequently derived from the oxygen molecule. To keep these in check under normal circumstances, a sophisticated system of protective mechanisms has evolved. Components of this system include vitamins E and C, beta-carotene and a number of enzymes which have at their active centre minerals such as selenium or zinc (see Table 10.9). In spite of the comprehensive system, free radicals do appear to leak from cells, albeit in minute amounts. These can attack and modify susceptible molecules such as the polyunsaturates (mainly linoleic acid) in LDL particles.

119

Under normal circumstances these molecules would be protected by antioxidants carried within the LDL particle, such as vitamin E. However, when antioxidant status is compromised — either because of poor dietary intake of these nutrients or because of high requirements, for example in smokers who are continually bombarding their lungs and other tissues with millions of free radicals in need of quenching — this protective mechanism will be impaired.

The susceptibility of the LDL particle depends, therefore, partly on its fatty acid composition, partly upon its own antioxidant status, and also upon its size (small particles are more susceptible). There is increasing evidence that particles enriched with monounsaturates by dietary means are relatively resistant to such damage (see Table 1, Part 1, page 12 for sources of fatty acids in the British diet).

These processes may help to explain why populations with high intakes of antioxidant vitamins and with a high proportion of monounsaturates in their diet tend to have lower standardized mortality rates for coronary heart disease. These processes may also help to explain some of the epidemiological findings which cannot be explained by the 'lipid hypothesis' alone.

High risk strategy versus population strategy

In Chapter 7 of Part 1, the main intervention strategies — the population (or public health) approach and the high risk approach — were discussed. The former approach aims to reduce the prevalence of coronary heart disease risk factors and subsequent disease incidence in the entire population via promotion of health-orientated changes in behaviour. The high risk strategy, on the other hand, focuses on identification and treatment of high risk individuals in order to reduce their risk factor levels. This latter approach is particularly well suited to primary health care.

A major limitation of the high risk approach is that most deaths from coronary heart disease do not occur among those at the top end of the distribution for any particular risk factor, for example the highest blood cholesterol levels. The distribution of blood cholesterol levels within a population at risk of coronary heart disease is so wide that the majority of deaths occur among those with moderate cholesterol concentrations. This is demonstrated by data from the Framingham Study (Figure 10.5). On the other hand, a limitation of the population approach is that many of those who will be in receipt of advice about a particular risk factor will already have low levels of that particular risk factor. However, some would agree that this does not matter because, as shown in Figure 10.5, the relationship between coronary heart disease mortality and blood cholesterol level is basically linear, with no evidence of a threshold level above which risk begins to exist (Lewis et al., 1986). The UK government argues that a population strategy is the only means of reaching the large number of people with modestly elevated levels of the major risk factors in whom the majority of deaths occur. Figure 10.5 also demonstrates why interventions should not focus on only one risk factor, coronary heart disease is a multi-factorial disease, and only about half of deaths from coronary heart disease can be attributed to high blood cholesterol levels, smoking and high blood pressure (see page 111).

Advantages of the high risk strategy are that the intervention is appropriate to the individual, who is likely to be motivated, but such an approach may not always be a cost-effective use of resources.

Advantages of the population approach are that it attempts to remove the underlying cause and has the potential to influence a far broader group of those at risk. However, there are disadvantages in that it offers only small benefits to the individual (see below) and this does not help to motivate the public or the health professional.

It has been argued that neither approach is acceptable on its own. Whilst it is important

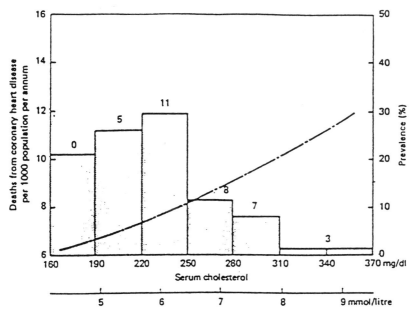

Figure 10.5 *Prevalence distribution (histogram) of serum cholesterol concentrations related to coronary heart disease mortality in men aged 55–64 years*
Source: Rose (1981). Reproduced with permission of the BMJ Publishing Group.

to treat those identified as at high risk, on a community basis this will have relatively little effect on death rates. Using data from population studies, it has been predicted that quite small reductions in the mean plasma cholesterol concentration of a population can result in quite substantial improvements in coronary death rates. Rose (1986) coined the phrase 'prevention paradox' to describe the phenomenon by which preventive actions that greatly benefit the population as a whole may bring only small benefits for individuals within that population. For example, Grover and colleagues (1994) have predicted that the benefit in life expectancy to individuals at moderate risk who follow dietary guidelines for fat reduction is no more than a matter of months whereas for smoking cessation, the benefits amount to an additional 2–4 years. The predicted population benefits in terms of coronary mortality associated with such interventions are considerably greater. This concept is central to any comparisons of the merits of high risk versus population strategies. If a large benefit is attained by a very few people (high risk strategy) then the population as a whole is not much better off.

However, if the prevalence of a risk factor is extensive, then relatively small improvements in this risk factor could amount to substantial population benefits. Rose (1981) described this as 'population-attributable risk' — the product of the risk for an individual and the prevalence of the risk within the population (see Figure 10.5).

Lewis et al. (1986) stressed the interdependency of the two strategies — the more effective the population strategy, the fewer people will require clinical care. When it comes to identification of those at high risk, there are two options — general population screening or opportunistic screening, for example routinely as part of any medical examination. The latter approach would seem the most realistic, but a cautious approach to the use of cholesterol-lowering drugs has been advocated (see page 103).

What can be done in practical terms?

Those working in general practice are in the

front line in terms of taking forward the Health of the Nation initiative and helping in the achievement of the targets. In Part 1, pages 23–26, ideas are given about how effective risk factor counselling can be conducted.

But the task will not be an easy one. Since publication of the targets, intakes of fat and saturates (as a proportion of food energy) have fallen marginally. But the Health Survey of Adults indicates that plasma cholesterol values have changed little since 1987, and since that time the proportion of adults who are overweight has been increasing steadily (OPCS, 1993; Bennett et al., 1995). The figures for obesity are particularly alarming.

So, much still needs to be done. Some recent reports (Robertson et al., 1992; Hunninghake et al., 1993) have suggested that dietary advice is ineffective in reducing plasma cholesterol to any significant degree in free-living healthy people. Yet in Finland they have managed to reduce the average for the whole population by more than 1 mmol/l. One explanation of these findings is that the dietary advice and mode of counselling given in the UK are at fault. It is essential that sound and comprehensive dietary advice is always given. Although there are not enough dietitians to make it feasible for them to provide routinely the dietary advice direct to the patient, dietitians can be used as a resource in the training of practice staff.

The importance of explanatory materials, regular contact, support and follow-up should not be under-estimated. Surveys have shown that the public still have great difficulty in translating healthy eating messages into food choices. We cannot expect patients to act effectively on advice as limited as 'eat more fibre', 'cut down on fat'. This advice needs to be translated for the majority of people **in the context of their current eating patterns.** Find out what they are eating currently before giving advice on what they should do in the future. People are more likely to be able to act on advice if it bears some relation to the foods they are choosing

at the time. Also, one should not be trapped into thinking that token changes (or token advice) will be adequate. To meet the targets set for fat, for example, all sources of fat in the diet will need consideration — not just the ones that are easy to change such as the type of milk. (See Part 1 for more information.)

The potential benefit of increased levels of activity should not be under-estimated. Apart from benefits to cardiovascular and skeletal fitness, increased physical activity will help people to balance their energy intake and so prevent weight gain and possibly also promote weight loss. Provided any additional energy needs are met via starchy high fibre foods, this approach will also benefit the ratio of calories derived from fat in the diet.

References

Anderson KM et al. (1991) An updated coronary risk profile: A statement for health professionals. *Circulation* **83,** 356–62.

Ascherio A et al. (1994) Trans fatty acids, intake and risk of myocardial infarction. *Circulation* **89,** 94–101.

Ashwell M (1991) Obesity in middle aged women. Proceedings of a conference: Social Status and Health. London, National Dairy Council.

Barker DJP et al. (1990). Fetal and placental size and risk of hypertension in adult life. *British Medical Journal* **301,** 259–62.

Barker DJP (1992) *Fetal and Infant Origins of Adult Disease.* London, British Medical Journal.

Barker DJP et al. (1993a) The relation of small head circumference and thinness at birth to death from cardiovascular disease in adult life. *British Medical Journal* **306,** 422–6.

Barker DJP et al. (1993b) Growth in utero and serum cholesterol concentrations in adult life. *British Medical Journal* **307,** 1524–7.

Bellizzi MC et al. (1994) Vitamin E and coronary heart disease: the European paradox. *European Journal of Clinical Nutrition* **48,** 822–31.

Bennett N et al. (1995) *Health Survey for England 1995.* London, Office of Population Censuses and Surveys.

British Nutrition Foundation (1987) *Task Force Report on Trans Fatty Acids.* London, BNF.

British Nutrition Foundation (1990) *Complex Carbohydrates in Food: the Report of the British Nutrition Foundation Task Force.* London, BNF.

British Nutrition Foundation (1993) *Coronary Heart Disease — 4.* London, BNF.

Brown A (1992) Oxidatively modified lipoproteins in coronary heart disease. *British Nutrition Foundation Bulletin* **17** (Suppl. 1), 49–64.

Burr M et al. (1989) Effects of changes in fat, fish and fibre intakes on death and myocardial infarction: diet and reinfarction trial (DART). *Lancet* **2**, 757–61.

Buttriss JL et al. (1991) *Coronary Heart Disease II. Fact File 8*. London, National Dairy Council.

Buttriss JL et al. (1993) *Coronary Heart Disease I (revised). Fact File 7*. London, National Dairy Council.

Charnock JS (1994) Dietary fats and cardiac arrhythmia in primates. *Nutrition* **19**, 161–9.

Davey-Smith G et al. (1993) Cholesterol lowering and mortality: the importance of considering initial levels of risk. *British Medical Journal* **305**, 1367–73.

Department of Health, Committee on Medical Aspects of Food Policy (1991) *Dietary Reference Values for Food Energy and Nutrients. Report on Health and Social Subjects 41*. London, HMSO.

Department of Health (1992) *Health of the Nation*. London, HMSO.

Department of Health, Committee on Medical Aspects of Food Policy (1994) *Nutritional Aspects of Cardiovascular Disease*. Report of the Cardiovascular Review Group. *Report on Health and Social Subjects 46*. London, HMSO.

Ernst E (1990) Plasma fibrinogen – an independent cardiovascular risk factor. *Journal of Internal Medicine* **227**, 365–72.

European Atherosclerosis Society (1992) *A Desk-top Guide to the Management of Risk Factors for Coronary Heart Disease*. EAS.

Fall CHD et al. (1992) Relation of infant feeding to adult serum cholesterol concentration and death from ischaemic heart disease. *British Medical Journal* **304**, 00–00.

Fleck A (1989) Latitude and ischaemic heart disease. *Lancet* **1**, 613.

Frankel EN et al. (1993) Inhibition of oxidation of human low density lipoprotein by phenolic substances in red wine. *Lancet* **341**, 454–7.

Gey KF (1986) On the antioxidant hypothesis with regard to arteriosclerosis. *Bibliotheca Nutrition Dieta* **37**, 53–91.

Gey KF et al. (1991) Inverse correlation between plasma vitamin E and mortality from ischaemic heart disease in cross-cultural epidemiology. *American Journal of Clinical Nutrition* **53**, 326S–334S.

Gregory J et al. (1990) *The Dietary and Nutritional Survey of British Adults*. London, HMSO.

Grobee DE et al. (1990) Coffee, caffeine and cardiovascular disease in men. *New England Journal of Medicine* **323**, 1026–32.

Grover SA et al. (1994) Life expectancy following dietary modification or smoking cessation. *Archives of Internal Medicine* **154**, 1696–1704.

Hales CN et al. (1991) Fetal and infant growth and impaired glucose tolerance at age 64. *British Medical Journal* **303**, 1019–22.

Hardman AE et al. (1989) Brisk walking and plasma high density lipoprotein cholesterol concentration in previously sedentary women. *British Medical Journal* **299**, 1204–5.

Health Education Authority (1990) *Health Update I: Coronary Heart Disease*. London, HEA.

Health Education Authority (1992) *Allied Dunbar National Fitness Survey*. London, HEA.

Hunninghake DB et al. (1993) The efficacy of intensive dietary therapy alone or combined with Lovastatin in outpatients with hypercholesterolaemia. *New England Journal of Medicine* **328**, 1213–9.

Jackson RL et al. (1984) Influence of polyunsaturated and saturated fats on plasma lipids and lipoproteins in man. *American Journal of Clinical Nutrition* **39**, 589–97.

Jackson R et al. (1991) Alcohol consumption and risk of coronary heart disease. *British Medical Journal* **303**, 211–6.

James WPT et al. (1989) The Mediterranean Diet: protective or simply non-toxic. *European Journal of Clinical Nutrition* **43** (Suppl. 2), 31–41.

Kohlmeier M et al. (1985) Influence of 'normal' and 'prudent' diets on biliary and serum lipids in healthy women. *American Journal of Clinical Nutrition* **42**, 1202–5.

Kwiterovitch PO et al. (1985) Effect of dietary treatment on the plasma levels of lipids, lipoprotein, cholesterol and LDL B protein in children with type ii hyperlipoproteinaemina. In *Detection and Treatment of Lipid and Lipoprotein Disorders in Childhood*. Ed. Wildhalm K and Nanto HK. New York, Alan R Liss. pp 123–7.

Lakka TA et al. (1994) Relation of leisure time physical activity and cardio-respiratory fitness to the risk of acute myocardial infarction in men. *New England Journal of Medicine* **330**, 1549–54.

Larsson B et al. (1992) Is abdominal body fat distribution a major explanation for the sex difference in the incidence of myocardial infarction? *American Journal of Epidemiology* **135**, 266–73.

Law MR et al. (1991) By how much does dietary salt reduction lower blood pressure? *British Medical Journal* **302**, 811–24.

Law MR et al. (1994a) Assessing possible hazards of reducing serum cholesterol. *British Medical Journal* **308**, 373–9.

Law MR et al. (1994b) By how much and how quickly does reduction in serum cholesterol concentration lower risk of ischaemic heart disease? *British Medical Journal* **308**, 367–73.

Lewis B et al. (1986) Reducing the risks of coronary heart disease in individuals and the population. *Lancet* **1**, 956–9.

Manson JE (1990) A prospective study of obesity

and risk of coronary heart disease in women. *New England Journal of Medicine* **322,** 882–9.

Marmot MG et al. (1978) Employment grade and coronary heart disease in British civil servants. *Journal of Epidemiology and Community Health* **32,** 244–9.

Mattson FH and Grundy SM (1985) Comparisons of the effects of dietary saturated, monosaturated and polyunsaturated fatty acids on plasma lipids and lipoproteins in man. *Journal of Lipid Research* **26,** 194–202.

McKeigue PM et al. (1991) Relation of central obesity and insulin resistance with high diabetes prevalence and cardiovascular risk in South Asians. *Lancet* **337,** 382–6.

Mensink RP and Katan MB (1990) Effect of dietary trans fatty acids on high density and low density lipoprotein cholesterol levels in healthy subjects. *New England Journal of Medicine* **323,** 439–45.

Mensink RP et al. (1992) Effect of dietary cis and trans fatty acids on serum lipoprotein (a) levels in humans. *Journal of Lipid Research* **33,** 1439–1501.

MRC Epidemiology Unit (1991) Epidemiological studies of cardiovascular disease. *Progress* Report VII.

Nestel P et al. (1992) Plasma lipoprotein lipid and Lp(a) changes with substitution of elaidic acid for oleic acid in the diet. *Journal of Lipid Research* **33,** 1029–36.

Office of Population Censuses and Surveys (1993) *Health Survey of England 1991.* London, HMSO.

Pancharuniti N et al. (1994) Plasma homocyst(e)ine, folate and vitamin B_{12} concentrations and risk of early-onset coronary artery disease. *American Journal of Clinical Nutrition* **59,** 940–8.

Pocock SJ et al. (1987) Social class differences in ischaemic heart disease. *British Medical Journal* **298,** 998–1002.

Puska P et al. (1985) Dietary fat and blood pressure; an intervention study on the effects of a low-fat diet with two levels of polyunsaturated fat. *Preventive Medicine* **14,** 573–84.

Pyörälä K et al. (1994) Prevention of coronary heart disease in clinical practice: Recommendations of the Task Force of the European Society of Cardiology, European Atherosclerosis Society and European Society of Hypertension. *Atherosclerosis* **110,** 121–61.

Renaud S and De Lorgeril M (1992) Wine, alcohol, platelets and the French paradox for coronary heart disease. *Lancet* **339,** 1523–6.

Renaud S et al. (1992) Alcohol and platelet aggregation; the Caerphilly prospective heart study. *American Journal of Clinical Nutrition* **55,** 1012–7.

Rimm EB et al. (1993) Vitamin E consumption and the risk of coronary heart disease in men. *New England Journal of Medicine* **328,** 1450–6.

Robertson I et al. (1992) Motivational effect of cholesterol measurement in general practice health checks. *British Journal of General Practice* **42,** 469–72.

Rose G (1981) Strategy of prevention; lessons from cardiovascular disease. *British Medical Journal* **282,** 1847–51.

Rose G (1986) Sick individuals and sick populations. *International Journal of Epidemiology* **14,** 32–38.

Salonen JT et al. (1991) Interactions of serum copper, selenium, and low density lipoprotein cholesterol in atherogenesis. *British Medical Journal* **302,** 756–60.

Seidelin KN et al. (1992) n-3 fatty acids in adipose tissue and coronary heart disease are inversely related. *American Journal of Clinical Nutrition* **55,** 1117–9.

Shaper AG et al. (1988) Alcohol and mortality in British men; explaining the U-shaped curve. *Lancet* **2,** 1267–73.

Stamler J et al. (1980) Prevention and control of hypertension by nutritional-hygienic means. Long-term experiences in the Chicago coronary prevention evaluation programme. *Journal of the American Medical Association* **243,** 1819–23.

Stampfer MJ et al. (1993) Vitamin E consumption and the risk of coronary heart disease in women. *New England Journal of Medicine* **328,** 1444–9.

Suadicani P et al. (1992) Serum selenium concentration and risk of ischaemic heart disease in a prospective cohort study of 3000 males. *Atherosclerosis* **96,** 33–42.

Troisi R et al. (1992) Trans fatty acid intake in relation to serum lipid concentration in adult men. *American Journal of Clinical Nutrition* **56,** 1019–1204.

Vartiainen E et al. (1994) Changes in risk factors explain changes in mortality from ischaemic heart disease in Finland. *British Medical Journal* **309,** 23–27.

Vartiainen E et al. (1995) Do changes in cardiovascular risk factors explain changes in mortality from stroke in Finland? *British Medical Journal* **310,** 901–4.

Wahle KWJ and James WPT (1993) Isometric fatty acids and human health. *European Journal of Clinical Nutrition* **47,** 828–39.

Wahle KWJ (1994) Are trans fatty acids in food deleterious to health? In *RCGP 1994 Members' Reference Book.* London, Sterling.

Willett WC et al. (1993) Intake of trans fatty acids and risk of coronary heart disease among women. *Lancet* **341,** 581–5.

11

Osteoporosis

Key points

1. Osteoporosis occurs when bone loss associated with the ageing process progresses to the extent that bones become sufficiently fragile to fracture.

2. It can be primary (postmenopausal and age-related forms), or secondary to underlying conditions or corticosteroid treatment.

3. It is most prevalent in postmenopausal women. It is estimated that more than 1 in 3 postmenopausal women have osteoporosis. In men the incidence is over 1 in 20.

4. There are two approaches to reducing the prevalence of osteoporosis — increasing peak bone mass at skeletal maturity, and slowing the rate of bone loss after the menopause and with ageing.

5. A healthy diet, incorporating calcium-rich foods, coupled with regular moderate exercise is thought to be important in maximizing peak bone mass during childhood and adolescence. Both factors can also help bone retain its strength throughout life. Smoking is detrimental to bone density.

6. Hormone replacement therapy is the most effective method of reducing post-menopausal bone loss. The role of additional calcium is controversial but the Department of Health advises that women at risk of osteoporosis may benefit from a diet richer in calcium than that proposed for the general population. For older people, in whom absorption may be impaired, the value of extra dietary calcium in improving calcium balance is more convincing, and adequate vitamin D intake is also important.

Loss of bone mass occurs as part of the ageing process. When this loss is excessive, osteoporosis results. In this condition, loss of trabecular and cortical bone is sufficient to lead to diminished physical strength of the skeleton and an increased susceptibility to fractures. It is conventional to classify osteoporosis as either primary or secondary:

- **Primary osteoporosis** includes post-menopausal and age-related forms and idiopathic osteoporosis of premenopausal women and young or middle-aged men. Bone loss accelerates in women for about five years after the menopause, occurring at a slower rate before and after (Parfitt, 1988). The menopausal acceleration is clearly related to a fall in circulating oestrogen levels.

- **Secondary osteoporosis** occurs as a result of an underlying condition such as rheumatoid disease, hyperthyroidism, chronic liver disease and intestinal malabsorption, or treatment such as corticosteroid therapy. It can also be associated with amenorrhoea and anorexia nervosa.

The incidence of hip fracture, considered to be closely associated with osteoporosis, has risen from 10 000 cases per year in the 1960s to almost 50 000 per year in the 1980s. The National Osteoporosis Society (1993) claims that not only has the incidence of hip fracture risen to 60 000 cases a year, causing 40 premature deaths each day, but spinal fractures are also increasing and are associated with premature death in a substantial proportion of osteoporosis sufferers.

More than 1 in 3 postmenopausal women and 1 in 20 men suffer pain and disability from fractures because their bones have become too porous and brittle (NOS, 1993). This incidence increases with age. In postmenopausal women, fractures are seen mainly as crush fractures of the vertebrae or wrist. In elderly people, fractures of the hip are more common.

Every year, the NHS spends more than £160 million on the direct hospital costs of treating hip fracture alone. When the cost for provision of social services and nursing care in the community are added, the bill rises to more than £640 million (NOS, 1993). These costs, however, say nothing about the pain, loss of mobility and independence, and ultimate isolation which osteoporosis can cause. More than half the elderly suffering a hip fracture each year will become dependent on relatives or friends or be confined to a nursing home for the rest of their life.

There are a number of inherited and environmental factors which have been associated with the risk of developing osteoporosis, such as race, gender, genetics, hormonal status, smoking and alcohol intake. Particularly important lifestyle factors are exercise and life-long dietary calcium intake (see below).

There are two approaches to the prevention of this disease: increasing peak bone mass at skeletal maturity and reducing the rate of bone loss after the menopause.

Peak bone mass

Bone is constantly turning over, a continuous process of resorption (bone breakdown) and formation. The majority of bone is formed during childhood and adolescence, the rate of deposition of bone minerals predominating over the rate of resorption. During the adolescent growth spurt, 45% of the adult skeletal size is formed (Matkovic, 1991). At this age, bone mineral content is increasing at the rate of about 8.5% per year.

Following adolescence, although bones no longer increase in length, they continue to increase in density during early adulthood. Hereditary factors are important in determining whether a person has a large or small bone mass. Both exercise and good overall

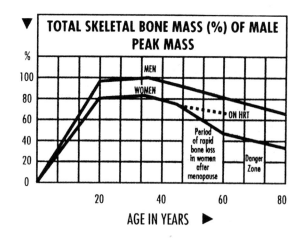

This diagram illustrates the average of what is believed to happen, although individuals may vary.

Figure 11.1 *Changes in bone mass with age*
Source: National Osteoporosis Society (1993).
MOT: Menopause and Osteoporosis Therapy.
Reproduced with permission of the publisher.

nutrition are important in this process. By the age of about 20 years, 90%–95% of the peak bone mass will have been achieved (DH, 1991).

In later life, resorption predominates over formation. Reduction in bone density begins at 35–40 years of age at a rate of about 0.3%–0.4% a year. The rate accelerates markedly for five years or more at the menopause (Figure 11.1). At the same time resorption is increased, exaggerating the existing bone imbalance. During this time, the yearly rate of bone loss may reach 5%.

Thus women may lose as much as 50% of their bone mass during a period of just 10 years around the time of the menopause, although average losses are less (Figure 11.1). If this rapid loss should occur relatively early because of an early natural menopause or because of surgical removal of the ovaries, the risk of becoming seriously osteoporotic will rise.

Calcium

Nearly all the calcium in the body (99%) is found in the skeleton. The remaining 1% of

Table 11.1 *Reference nutrient intakes for calcium*

Age	mg/day
0–12 months	525
1–3 years	350
4–6 years	450
7–10 years	550
Males	
11–14 years	1000
15–18 years	1000
19–50 years	700
50+ years	700
Females★	
11–14 years	800
15–18 years	800
19–50 years	700
50+ years	700
Lactation (increments)	
0–4 months	+ 550
5+ months	+ 550

★There is no longer an increment for pregnant women. This assumes women enter pregnancy adequately nourished.
Source: Department of Health (1991).

Table 11.2 *Typical calcium content of foods*

$^1/_3$ pint (190 ml) semi-skimmed milk	231 mg
$^1/_3$ pint (190 ml) skimmed milk	236 mg
$^1/_3$ pint (190 ml) whole (silver top) milk	225 mg
1 oz (28 g) Cheddar or other hard cheese	207 mg
5 oz (140 g) pot of yogurt	240 mg
3 oz (84 g) cottage cheese	60 mg
2 oz (60 g) fromage frais	53 mg
4 oz (112 g) ice-cream	134 mg
2 tablespoons (30 g) single cream	27 mg
2 oz (56 g) canned sardines in tomato sauce (including bones)	230 mg
2 large slices (60 g) white bread	66 mg
2 large slices (60 g) wholemeal bread	32 mg
4 oz (112 g) spring cabbage	34 mg
4 oz (112 g) broccoli	85 mg
4 oz (112 g) baked beans	50 mg
2 oz (56 g) peanuts	34 mg
2 oz (56 g) dried apricots	52 mg
1 large orange	58 mg
3 oz (84 g) shelled prawns	126 mg
1 egg (50 g)	29 mg

body calcium is found in extracellular fluids, intracellular structures and cell membranes. Levels of soft tissue calcium, particularly blood levels of ionized calcium, are maintained at the expense of bone in the face of inadequate calcium intake or absorption. A regular dietary supply of calcium is essential and it is absorbed predominantly in the small intestine. The calcium requirement of an individual is the amount necessary to maintain calcium balance.

The UK reference nutrient intakes (DH, 1991), which include a safety margin over and above requirement and so should be sufficient for the needs of about 97% of the population group to which they refer, are given in Table 11.1 (more information about UK dietary reference values can be found in Part 1, Appendix 2). Dietary sources of calcium are given in Table 11.2.

The dietary reference values adopted by different countries vary. Typically, those adopted in the USA are higher than in Britain and a number of other countries, and consistent with this, the UK reference values for calcium are lower than those which exist in the USA. Nevertheless, since the British dietary reference values were established, various studies have been published which support the higher values adopted in the States (see page 128). The British reference values are unlikely to be reviewed before the end of the decade, and there is no certainty that British scientists will see the need to follow the American lead. What remains certain is the requirement for young people in particular to maintain good intakes of dietary calcium to meet their needs (see Chapter 4) and optimize the calcification of their bones.

Childhood and adolescence

The higher recommendations for calcium in older children and adolescents compared with adults reflect the amounts required during the growing period for optimal calcification of the skeleton. Peak bone mass appears to be related to intake of calcium (and physical activity level) during the years of bone remineralization.

In Britain, reference values fall to adult levels at age 18 years. However, in the USA, the higher recommendation of 1200 mg of calcium per day (see page127) is retained into early adulthood and applies to those aged 11–24 years (National Research Council, 1989). This reflects American views, which differ from those in Britain, on the quantities of calcium needed by children, adolescents and young adults in order to ensure optimal bone calcification. In the light of new information, some scientists in the USA are still not content with these higher levels, set in 1989. A US National Institute of Health Consensus Development Conference (Rowe, 1994) has suggested that intakes in this age group should be even higher — 1500 mg — and that intakes in those aged 1–10 years should be 1200 mg instead of the current US recommendation of 800 mg.

Lee and colleagues (1993), studying pre-school children, have reported that calcium intake during the period from birth to five years showed a significant and positive correlation with bone mineral content at age five. Calcium intake in the second year of life appeared particularly important.

Matkovic et al. (1990) carried out a study in 14-year-old girls which was designed to evaluate the need for calcium during adolescence, to assess the effect of mineral supplementation on bone mass, and to evaluate the possible genetic influence on bone status. Results indicated that adolescent girls were able to retain 200–400 mg of calcium per day provided sufficient was available in the diet. Since absorption of a given dose of calcium is incomplete and there are obligatory daily calcium losses of 150 mg or more per day, this level of accretion translates into an intake of up to 1800 mg daily, according to Matkovic. Intakes below 500 mg/day may translate into inadequate calcium and increased risk of osteoporosis in later life. There was a more pronounced increase in bone mass over time in the calcium-supplemented group (1640 mg calcium/day) than in the control group (average of 750 mg calcium/day) but the differences between bone mass measurements were not statistically significant. By 16 years of age, daughters had accumulated 90%–97% of the bone mass of their premenopausal mothers.

In another study of teenagers, bone mineral density of the femoral neck continued to increase up to calcium intakes of 1200 mg per day, at which point no further increase was seen (Valimaki et al., 1994).

The higher the bone mass at skeletal maturity, the better prepared will be the skeleton for later bone loss. Regular exercise favours calcium accumulation and this leads to stronger bones. Armstrong et al. (1990) have shown that children are taking less exercise, which may have an important impact on maximizing the genetic potential for bone mass. For girls, relative oestrogen deficiency has a negative effect on bone mass. This includes late menarche, very irregular menstruation, and amenorrhoea, which may, for example, occur with regular excessive exercise and/or anorexia nervosa (see Chapters 4 and 9). Valimaki and colleagues' study (1994) indicates that calcium intake, exercise and not smoking are all factors which promote improved bone density in adolescents and young adults.

Adults

Despite the fact that adult height (and closure of the epiphyseal plates) is reached in adolescence, the need for calcium does not cease. Bone is a living dynamic tissue, which is constantly being repaired and replaced throughout life by a process that involves continuous movement of calcium between bone and blood. During the third decade of life calcium accretion and the consequent increase in bone density both continue. After this time, however, resorption begins to outstrip formation (Figure 11.1).

Exercise as well as abstinence from tobacco and moderation in alcohol intake may also be beneficial for the skeleton (Stevenson et al., 1989; Hernandez-Avila et al., 1991). Heavy smoking can induce menopause up to five years earlier and has a suppressive effect on bone building cells (osteoblasts). Passive smokers are also affected and have their menopause three years earlier, on average (NOS, 1993).

Postmenopause

Oestrogen has a protective effect on the bone, but ovarian production ceases at the menopause. Consequently its loss results in a relatively rapid loss in bone for a few years after the menopause, after which time bone loss reverts to its previous rate (Figure 11.1). Oestrogens continue to be produced in small quantities in adipose tissue, however, which may in part explain the relative susceptibility of underweight women to osteoporosis. Although calcium is required throughout life there is conflicting evidence as to whether **extra** calcium at the time of the menopause can be of benefit. The consensus seems to be that there is little evidence that extra calcium can actually prevent the increased loss of bone density resulting from lack of oestrogen seen in post-menopausal women immediately after the menopause (Riggs et al., 1987; Stevenson et al., 1988).

However, there is more evidence of a benefit in women five or more years past the menopause. A recent study (Reid et al., 1993) has confirmed earlier findings such as those of Dawson-Hughes et al. (1990) that calcium supplementation can significantly slow bone loss in both the spine and the limbs in normal postmenopausal women. Furthermore, it is not necessary for calcium intake to have been previously low for the benefits to be seen. Nevertheless, women who have a low intake of calcium may benefit, in particular, from an improved dietary intake or supplementation (Dawson-Hughes et al., 1990).

More than 40 studies with postmenopausal women have been reviewed recently by Heaney (1993). He concluded that in the 19 studies which controlled for calcium intake, additional calcium was shown to slow or stop bone loss; and in each of 14 studies which excluded women who had recently passed the menopause, a benefit of extra calcium was seen. Heaney is clearly convinced that for such women, extra calcium can be of benefit, but it is as yet unclear how much should be advised. He also believes that vitamin D is important (see page 130).

Two recent European studies in elderly people have shown that it is never too late to start treatment with vitamin D, and fracture rates can fall in as little as 18 months (Chapuy et al., 1992; Heikineimo et al., 1992).

Some work has indicated that smaller amounts of hormone replacement therapy (HRT) are needed when calcium intakes are high (Ettinger et al., 1987). The Department of Health (1991) did not believe it necessary to advise higher intakes of calcium for post-menopausal women. However, it has indicated that for those who are considered to be at high risk of osteoporosis, a diet richer in calcium than that advocated for the general population might be prudent.

Use of hormone replacement therapy

It is clear that appropriate doses of oestrogens are effective in reducing or completely suppressing postmenopausal bone loss (Al-Azzawa et al., 1987; Kiel et al., 1987). It is most beneficial just after the menopause but studies have shown that use of oestrogens for at least 5 years after the menopause reduces the risk of hip and wrist fractures (Weiss et al., 1980; Pagamini-Hill et al., 1981). In one of these studies patients who used oestrogen for 6 years or more had halved their risk of subsequent fracture (Weiss et al., 1980). They conclude that there is a 20% reduction in osteoporotic fractures during the first 5 years of treatment and a 60% reduction after 5 years.

HRT has also been shown to decrease the risk of coronary heart disease (Bush, 1991) and stroke and to reduce the symptoms associated with the menopause. Unopposed oestrogen decreases total cholesterol, LDL-cholesterol and raises HDL-cholesterol. Recent work suggests that the addition of progestogens may not detract from this effect (NOS, 1993). But some questions have also been raised about its safety in relation to cancer. Patients taking HRT for more than 10 years need to be advised that there may be a slightly increased risk of breast cancer with long-term therapy. Some studies have shown an increased incidence, while others have not, and the apparent increase may be attributable to improved surveillance of women on HRT (Studd, 1992).

Unopposed oestrogen given to women with an intact uterus increases the risk of endometrial hyperplasia and endometrial carcinoma. But combining the oestrogen with a suitable dose of progestogen decreases the risk of endometrial carcinoma to a level less than that experienced by postmenopausal women not on HRT (Sturdee et al., 1978, Collins et al., 1980). HRT is not associated with increased risk of cervical cancer or cancer of the ovary (Hunt et al., 1987).

The National Osteoporosis Society (1993) suggests that on balance, not taking HRT seems to be riskier than taking it. This decision takes no account, though, of the cost of prescribing HRT routinely. The balance is further improved in favour of HRT if women particularly at risk of osteoporosis or coronary heart disease are considered in isolation. The balance is particularly in favour of women who have had a hysterectomy and are taking continuous oestrogen.

All women approaching the menopause should be encouraged to discuss HRT with their general practitioner or practice nurse. They may want to know about their personal risk before deciding. If DEXA (dual energy x-ray absorptiometry) scans are not available on the NHS locally, some women may choose to have a scan done privately.

Elderly

In elderly people, bone density is usually considerably reduced and it is likely that the absorption of calcium is less efficient. Vitamin D is required for the absorption of calcium,

and vitamin D status itself may also be poor because of malabsorption or gastric surgery, or as a result of abnormal hepatic metabolism (for example because of anticonvulsant therapy or liver disease). In addition, vitamin D synthesis via the exposure of skin to sunlight, the major source of vitamin D for most people, may also be reduced in those with reduced mobility or in those who are institutionalized and so unable to get out into the sunshine so frequently.

Typical intake of vitamin D from diet is 2 μg/day and the Department of Health recommends that housebound and institutionalized elderly people should receive a supplement to bring their daily intake up to 10 μg/day (DH, 1992). This can be provided as a daily supplement or as a six-monthly or annual depot injection.

However, for those who are able to get out into the sunshine, it has been demonstrated that limited exposure (hands, forearms and face) to even short periods of summer sunshine in May to September (15–30 minutes per day) can supply adequate amounts of vitamin D (Holick, 1990). Even dappled sunlight will be sufficient. Good dietary sources should also be encouraged (see Part 1, page 45).

Several studies conducted among very elderly people have indicated the importance of adequate vitamin D status in the prevention of osteoporosis (for example, Chapuy et al., 1992).

In the British diet almost 60% of the average calcium intake from household food, a total of about 814 mg a day, comes from milk and its products (MAFF, 1994); 40% alone comes from milk. In this context, the recent COMA report on nutrition and elderly people noted the importance of the doorstep delivery service in enabling elderly people in particular to maintain their calcium intake (DH, 1992). A number of other foods also provide calcium (Table 11.2). However, in the absence of dairy products, these individually may not be included in the diet in sufficient quantities to meet calcium needs.

There are also differences between foods in the 'availability' of the calcium to the body. Calcium in dairy produce has a high bio-availability and is relatively easily absorbed in the intestine. This process is further assisted by the lactose and casein in milk. However, the calcium in other foods is not always so 'available' because co-existing food components restrict its absorption to varying extents. This is particularly the case for foods rich in dietary fibre and associated substances such as phytate and oxalate. The National Osteoporosis Society has a useful recipe booklet with information on calcium in the diet (free of charge to members).

Consequently, the importance of calcium and, in particular, vitamin D for this age group, as part of a balanced diet, should be emphasized.

Calcium absorption and calcium status

The following factors affect calcium absorption and calcium status:

Vitamin D is important for the absorption of calcium and for normal bone mineralization and metabolism. But there is little evidence that poor vitamin D status is causative in osteoporosis. However, as the main source of vitamin D results from the action of sunlight on skin, encouraging the intake of foods rich in this vitamin, together with supplements where appropriate, may be of benefit to elderly people who are housebound (see Part 1, Appendix 2 for foods rich in vitamin D; see also page 130).

Salt and sodium intake: High intakes of sodium are known to increase calcium excretion and although there is an adaptive response, this may be impaired in the elderly.

Fibre: A very high intake may reduce the bioavailability of calcium. However, it is not known if this is significant in the long term, as adaptation to high fibre intakes may occur. Raw bran is not recommended as this is known to reduce the absorption of a number of essential nutrients including calcium.

High protein diets: These have been related to a negative calcium balance. The level of protein in most British diets should not be a cause for concern, but the Department of Health (1991) suggests that protein intakes greater than twice the reference nutrient intake (1.5 g protein/kg body weight/day) are inappropriate.

Alcohol: Alcoholism accelerates bone loss, and in addition chronic alcoholics are likely to have a poor nutrient intake, accentuating the effect of the risk factor.

Exercise: In general, exercise is thought to be beneficial to the skeleton, with increased bone mass and strength occurring as a response to the increased mechanical load and stress on the skeleton, specifically in load-bearing bones. However, studies of female high performance long-distance runners and ballet dancers have found that these individuals may have reduced bone mass (Wolman et al., 1992). Many young female athletes are amenorrhoeic as a result of intensive training programmes. Dietary intake may also be inadequate. Since the implications of such practices for future bone health are not known, it would seem prudent to advocate realistic training programmes and a sensible balanced diet (see Appendix 1 and Part 1, page 31) for young people, particularly when growth is still underway.

Opportunities for prevention

As part of the Department of Health's new health promotion programmes, general practitioners are encouraged to target groups in the practice population who might benefit from health promotion interventions.

Opportunities for health promotion in relation to the prevention of osteoporosis exist via general health promotion of the benefits of a good diet and plenty of exercise, opportunistic counselling, identification of individuals at risk, well woman/contraception advice/menopause clinics, group education of cohorts of women (for example targeted through age/sex registers). Table 11.3 provides suggestions regarding appropriate

Table 11.3 *Ideas which may help in the prevention of osteoporosis*

Age group	Normal policy	Special risk factors to look for
Children, adolescents, young adults	Encourage good nutrition, calcium-rich foods, plenty of exercise Discourage smoking and high alcohol intake	Anorexia nervosa, persistent amenorrhoea, heavy smoker, early menopause (natural, surgical), vegan, lactose intolerant, generally poor diet
Menopausal women	The above Discuss HRT	Family history of early osteoporosis, early menopause, history of poor diet, vegan, lactose intolerant, heavy smoker, oral steroids, poor mobility, medical conditions which might provoke secondary osteoporosis
Postmenopausal women	The above Consider a bone scan depending on the presence of risk factors	The above Loss of height, back pain, previous fracture after minimal trauma

policy for three different age groups of women, together with particular risk factors which may necessitate more intensive action.

The National Osteoporosis Society's (1993) publication, *MOT: Menopause and Osteoporosis Therapy*, provides comprehensive advice for general practitioners and practice nurses on practical action that can be taken, including information on the various treatments available.

References

Al-Azzawa F et al. (1987) Long term effect of oestrogen therapy on bone mass as measured by duel photon absorptiometry. *British Medical Journal* **294**, 1261–2.

Armstrong N et al. (1990) Patterns of physical activity among 11–16 year old British children. *British Medical Journal* **301**, 203–5.

Bush TL (1991) Extra skeletal effects of oestrogen and prevention of atherosclerosis. *Osteoporosis International* **2**, 5–11.

Chapuy MC et al. (1992) Vitamin D₃ and calcium to prevent hip fractures in elderly women. *New England Journal of Medicine* **327**, 1637–42.

Collins J et al. (1980) Oestrogen use and survival in endometrial cancer. *Lancet* **2**, 961–4.

Dawson-Hughes B et al. (1990) A controlled trial of the effect of calcium supplementation on bone density in postmenopausal women. *New England Journal of Medicine* **324**, 878–83.

Department of Health, Committee on Medical Aspects of Food Policy (1991) *Dietary Reference Values for Food Energy and Nutrients for the United Kingdom. Report on Health and Social Subjects 41.* London, HMSO.

Department of Health, Committee on Medical Aspects of Food Policy (1992) *The Nutrition of Elderly People. Report on Health and Social Subjects 43.* London, HMSO.

Ettinger B et al. (1987) Postmenopausal bone loss is prevented by treatment with low dosage oestrogen with calcium. *Annals of Internal Medicine* **106**, 40–45.

Heaney RP (1993) Nutritional factors in osteoporosis. *Annual Reviews of Nutrition* **13**, 287–316.

Heikineimo RJ et al. (1992) Annual injection of vitamin D and fractures of aged bones. *Calcified Tissue International* **51**, 105–10.

Hernandez-Avila M et al. (1991) Caffeine, moderate alcohol intake, and risk of fractures of the hip and forearm in middle-age women. *American Journal of Clinical Nutrition* **54**, 157–63.

Holick MF (1990) The intimate relationship between the sun, skin and vitamin D: a new perspective.

Bone: Clinical and Biochemical News and Reviews **7,** 66–69.

Hunt K et al. (1987) Long term surveillance of mortality and cancer incidence in women receiving hormone replacement therapy. *British Journal of Obstetrics and Gynaecology and Reproductive Biology* **20,** 1–6.

Kiel D et al. (1987) Hip fractures and the use of oestrogen in postmenopausal women. *New England Journal of Medicine* **317,** 119–74.

Lee WTF et al. (1993) Relationship between long-term calcium intake and bone mineral content of children aged from birth to five years. *British Journal of Nutrition* **70,** 235–48.

Matkovic V (1991) Calcium metabolism and calcium requirements during skeletal modelling and consolidation of bone mass. *American Journal of Clinical Nutrition* **54,** 245S–260S.

Matkovic V et al. (1990) Factors that influence peak bone mass formation: a study of calcium balance and the inheritance of bone mass in adolescent females. *American Journal of Clinical Nutrition* **52,** 878–88.

Ministry of Agriculture, Fisheries and Food (1994) *Household Food Consumption and Expenditure 1993.* London, HMSO.

National Osteoporosis Society (1993) *MOT: Menopause and Osteoporosis Therapy.* Bath, National Osteoporosis Society.

National Research Council (1989) *Recommended Dietary Allowances.* 10th edn. Washington DC, National Academy of Sciences.

Pagamini-Hill A et al. (1981) Menopausal oestrogen therapy and hip fractures. *Annals of Internal Medicine* **95,** 28–31.

Parfitt AM (1988) Bone remodelling: relationships to the amount and structure of bone and the pathogenesis and prevention of fractures. In Riggs NL and Melton LJ (Eds) *Osteoporosis: Etiology, Diagnosis and Management.* New York, Rowen Press.

Reid R et al. (1993) Effects of calcium supplementation on bone loss in postmenopausal women. *New England Journal of Medicine* **328,** 460–4.

Riggs BL et al. (1987) Dietary calcium intake and rates of bone loss in women. *Journal of Clinical Investigation* **80,** 979–82.

Rowe PM (1994) New US recommendations on calcium intake. *Lancet* **343,** 1559–60.

Stevenson JC et al. (1988) Dietary intake of calcium and postmenopausal bone loss. *British Medical Journal* **297,** 15–17.

Stevenson JC et al. (1989) Determinants of bone density in normal women: risk factors for fracture osteoporosis. *British Medical Journal* **298,** 924–8.

Studd JWW (1992) Complications of oestrogen therapy in postmenopausal women. *Journal of the Royal Society of Medicine* **85,** 376–8.

Sturdee DW et al. (1978) Relations between bleeding pattern, endometrial histology, and oestrogen treatment in the postmenopausal woman. *British Medical Journal* **1,** 1575–7.

Valimaki MJ et al. (1994) Exercise, smoking and calcium intake during adolescence and early adulthood as determinants of peak bone mass. *British Medical Journal* **309,** 230–5.

Weiss NS et al. (1980) Decreased risk of fractures of the hip and lower forearm with the postmenopausal use of oestrogen. *New England Journal of Medicine* **303,** 1195–8.

Wolman RL et al. (1992) Dietary calcium as a statistical determinant of spinal trabecular bone density in amenorrhoeic and oestrogen-replete athletes. *Bone and Mineral* **17,** 415–23.

Further reading

Buttriss J and Gray J (1992) *Calcium and Health. Fact File 1.* London, NDC.

Christiansen C and Riis BJ (1990) *The Silent Epidemic. Postmenopausal Osteoporosis. A Handbook for the Medical Profession.* Bath, National Osteoporosis Society and European Foundation for Osteoporosis and Bone Disease.

Coope J (1989) *Hormone Replacement Therapy.* London, Royal College of General Practitioners.

Woolf AD and Dixon A (1988) *Osteoporosis: A Clinical Guide.* London, Martin Dunitz.

12

Weight management

Key points

1. The preferred method for assessing whether underweight or overweight exists is the body mass index.

2. There has been an increase in the prevalence of overweight and obesity during the last decade. This has led to a shift in emphasis towards prevention of overweight, especially among young adults, rather than only treating existing overweight and obesity.

3. Excess body weight carries health risks, which increase with the degree of obesity.

4. The risk to health is greater if the excess fat is mainly distributed around the central part of the body. This indicates an excess of internal fat and is associated with a predisposition towards coronary heart disease, stroke, diabetes, breast cancer and gallstones.

5. The practice team can play a key role in efforts to stop the increase and reduce the prevalence of overweight, but it is important to target endeavours.

6. Specialist knowledge is needed when advising overweight children and their parents about diet in relation to body weight.

7. Current research does not support a marked difference in eating behaviour between overweight and normal weight people.

8. The recommended type of slimming programme combines regular moderate physical activity with a reduced energy diet comprising a wide range of foods.

9. Very low calorie diets (VLCD) are designed to produce rapid weight loss. They should be used only if conventional methods have failed and they are not suitable for people with a relatively small amount of weight to be lost.

10. The plight of those trying to gain weight is often overlooked. Again, advice should be based on choices from the four main food groups. Inclusion of nutritious snacks can be helpful.

11. Specialist knowledge is required when advising patients suspected of having anorexia or bulimia nervosa.

Assessment of body weight

Although relative height for weight is still often used to assess whether a patient is overweight, the preferred method is the body mass index (or Quetelet index). This is the ratio of weight (kilograms) over the square of height (metres):

$$\frac{\text{Weight}}{(\text{Height})^2}$$

For example, the body mass index for a 70 kg man, 1.7 metres tall would be:

$$\frac{70}{1.7 \times 1.7} = 24.2$$

Table 12.1 gives the recommended classification of body weight according to the body mass index.

This method is applicable to adult men and women. However, it does not take body composition into consideration. Therefore, it may be inappropriate for certain people:

- children or adolescents (males and females under 18 years of age) as growth is still occurring. Tables of reference

Table 12.1 *Classification of body weight by body mass index*

Body mass index	Classification	Grade of obesity
Under 20	Underweight	
20–24.9	Normal weight	Grade 0
25–29.9	Overweight ('plump')	Grade I
30–40	Moderate obesity	Grade II
over 40	Severe obesity	Grade III

Source: Garrow (1988).

- pregnant women, owing to the growth of the developing baby and maternal stores

- individuals with a high proportion of muscle; those who take part in many sporting activities may appear to be in the overweight category when body mass index is calculated.

For convenience, the graph shown in Figure 12.1 can be used with patients in the age range 20–65 years. Suitable BMI ranges for children are being considered.

standard weights for children can be found in the report on dietary reference values (DH, 1991) and new centile charts for children have been developed (see page 22)

- elderly people, owing to the changes which occur in body composition as part of the natural ageing process

Prevalence of overweight

Overweight and obesity are among the commonest preventable health problems in the UK. However, the proportion of people classed as overweight or obese has increased in both men and women in Britain, during the last decade, as outlined in Table 12.2.

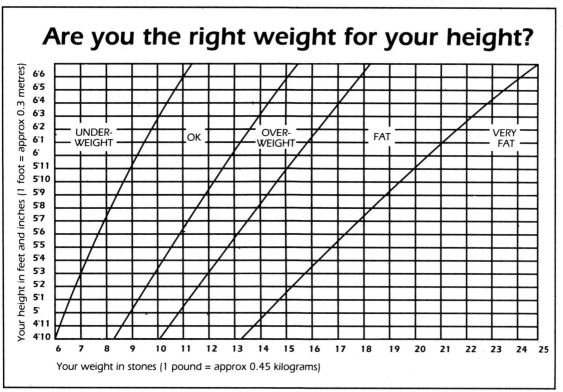

Figure 12.1 *The right weight for your height.*
Source: Health Education Authority (1991) *Enjoy Healthy Eating.* London, HEA. Reproduced with permission of the publisher.

Table 12.2 *Prevalence of overweight and obesity in Great Britain*

	1980 %	1987 %	1991 %	1993 %
Men				
Overweight/obese (BMI >25)	39	45	53	57
Obese (BMI >30)	6	8	13	13
Women				
Overweight/obese (BMI >25)	32	36	44	48
Obese (BMI >30)	8	12	16	16

Sources: Gregory et al. (1990); White et al. (1993); Bennett et al. (1995).

The Health of the Nation initiative aims to reduce the proportion of men and women aged 16–64 who are obese to no more than 6% (men) and 8% (women), by the year 2005 (see Part 1, page 2). Achievement of this appears increasingly unlikely (Table 12.2).

Health risks of excess weight

The health risks increase with the amount of excess weight carried. Obese people have a higher risk than lean people of developing hypertension, diabetes mellitus, hypercholesterolaemia (and hence cardiovascular disease), respiratory disease, certain forms of cancer, and gall stones. Obesity also aggravates some pre-existing conditions such as osteoarthritis of weight-bearing joints, and presents a risk for those undergoing surgery.

Health risks among those people who are merely overweight depend largely on age. Young overweight people (BMI of 25–30) are at risk in that they may well progress to becoming obese as they get older. They are especially at risk if there is a family history of hypertension and/or diabetes, in which case they have a 10% greater chance of premature death than people of the same age but of normal weight. In older people, for example over 50 years, being overweight (BMI of 25–30) does not seem to carry an **excess** mortality risk, although it may aggravate conditions such as osteoarthritis. Among obese people (BMI of 30 or over) mortality rates increase

with the degree of overweight, attributable largely to deaths from cardiovascular disease and non-insulin dependent diabetes. It has been estimated that the mortality rate of people with a BMI of 35 is about twice that of people of normal weight of the same age.

Fat distribution

The distribution of adipose tissue varies widely between individuals, with obvious characteristic differences between men and women. There is growing evidence to suggest that the specific distribution may be an additional influence on the health risks arising from obesity (Ashwell, 1992; Larsson et al., 1992; Wing, 1992).

The metabolic abnormalities associated with obesity, such as hyperlipidaemia and hyperinsulinaemia, and conditions such as diabetes and cardiovascular disease, are more closely linked with fat deposition that is relatively 'central' (around the waist) rather than that which is relatively 'peripheral' (around the hips and thighs). A greater amount of fat in the abdominal wall, close to the major organs, may be specifically related to the metabolic complications of obesity. The health risks associated with peripheral fat distribution tend to be related to the mechanical strain of carrying too much fat, for example varicose veins.

Fat distribution is measured by the waist to hip circumference ratio (WHR). A high ratio indicates central fat distribution (apple shape) whereas a low ratio indicates peripheral fat distribution (pear shape).

New approach to weight management

Traditionally, the approach taken in weight management has been to provide dietary advice to those patients who are already overweight or obese, occasionally also including specific advice on taking more exercise.

Clearly, this approach is not satisfactory since

the prevalence of overweight and obesity is progressively rising (Table 12.2).

A new approach is therefore needed and this has led to a shift in focus towards prevention of people becoming overweight in the first place. Furthermore, dietary modification is now being seen as inadequate in isolation and through the Physical Activity Task Force of the Health of the Nation initiative, consideration is now being given to ways of encouraging more physical activity in the lives of the population as a whole.

Treating those who are already obese will continue to be necessary, but it should be in the context of a growing awareness that periodic dieting is not the answer and that more fundamental changes in eating patterns and attitudes to physical activity are needed before there is a real likelihood of the Health of the Nation obesity targets being reached (see pages 135–7).

The primary health care team has a key role to play in assisting this process.

Macronutrient composition

In recent years attention has focused more closely on the role of macronutrient composition in weight management and it has been suggested that the composition of the diet may be important in promoting overeating. It has been assumed that one calorie from fat that is excess to requirements has the same potential to result in an increase in body weight as one calorie derived from carbohydrate. However, a number of studies now suggest that, calorie for calorie, fat is potentially more 'fattening' than carbohydrate, and that a high fat diet predisposes to overweight and obesity independently of total energy intake, partly by influencing appetite control (Prewitt et al., 1991; Sheppard et al., 1991; Tremblay et al., 1991, Bolton-Smith and Woodward, 1993).

It appears that weight maintenance is likely to be determined primarily by events pertaining to the metabolism of carbohydrate and fat (Flatt, 1987; Jéquier, 1994). Protein metabolism is virtually disregarded in this respect because it makes only a small contribution to total energy intake. In addition, protein balance tends to be maintained spontaneously even on diets of very diverse composition, provided that adequate amounts of protein are supplied.

In order to maintain a steady body weight, the average composition of the fuel mix (nutrients available in the body for energy metabolism) oxidized by the body must be the same as that of the nutrients supplied by the food eaten. In these conditions protein balance, carbohydrate balance and fat balance would be achieved (Tremblay et al., 1991). In obese people, there appears to be little or no ability in the short term to increase fat oxidation in response to excessive fat intakes in an attempt to burn off the excess. Instead, fat stores, the extent of which are virtually limitless, increase. By contrast, when intake of carbohydrate exceeds requirements, the excess is oxidized readily and in preference to fat (Flatt et al., 1985; Jéquier, 1994).

There is also evidence that spontaneous adjustments in food intake can occur in order to achieve carbohydrate balance (Jéquier, 1994). In the longer term, fat oxidation adapts to the higher body fat composition to bring fat intake and oxidation into equilibrium resulting in the maintenance of body fat stores at a new stable weight. Volschenk and colleagues (1993) suggest that, in obese people, the failure to increase fat oxidation in response to a raised intake may be due to higher levels of circulating free fatty acids which may mask the fat intake.

In summary, provided energy intake is in line with energy expenditure, body weight can be regulated over a wide range of fat to carbohydrate ratios (Hill and Prentice, 1995). However, when energy intake exceeds output, a diet high in fat is thought more likely to predispose to weight gain; in part because its high energy density (calories/g food) encourages overconsumption and in part because fat as a source of calories is spared relative to carbohydrate, encouraging deposition of fat in adipose tissue.

Alcohol and energy balance

The limited information available suggests that people do not compensate for energy taken in the form of alcohol by subsequently reducing energy intake from other sources, particularly when alcohol is consumed in the evening (DeCastro and Orozco, 1991). Furthermore, alcohol has been suggested to promote fat storage by being oxidized preferentially (Suter et al., 1992; Hill and Prentice, 1995).

Preventing obesity

It is likely that attempts to reduce the numbers of people who become overweight or who progress from overweight to obesity will be more effective if efforts are directed towards specific groups of the population. For example, the following groups could be targeted or supported by primary health care team members:

- children and adolescents, especially those who are already overweight or who have a family history of obesity (see below)

- those who have already lost weight but were previously obese

- people who are trying to give up smoking (see page 139)

- patients on prescribed drugs associated with weight gain.

Children and adolescents

Approximately 5% of children are overweight at the age of seven, with a bias towards girls. This figure increases to 9% by the age of 11 (Braddon et al., 1986). However, attempts to predict adult obesity from the presence of excess weight in childhood have been unsuccessful, especially when fatness is assessed in infancy and before five years of age.

Garrow (1991) proposes that there should be a policy in primary schools to identify overweight children because it seems that the problem is best tackled between the ages of seven and twelve years. He acknowledges that

this would require the co-operation of parents, school teachers, community dietitians, school nurses and caterers, as well as the primary health care team. Any attempts to normalize a child's body weight should be done in the context of the family unit, rather than singling out the child in isolation. This is particularly important in relation to the child's self-esteem. In many cases other family members will also benefit from advice on diet and exercise.

The nutrient density of a weight reduction diet for overweight and obese children who are still growing must be carefully considered. It is generally considered more appropriate to aim for maintenance of the current weight rather than weight loss, whilst growth in height continues. In addition to advice on diet, the importance of physical activity should also be stressed. The management of obesity in children is covered in more detail in Chapter 4.

There is currently much concern about the low reported levels of physical activity among children. Armstrong et al. (1990) have reported surprisingly low levels of physical activity in British children — many seldom experience the intensity and duration of physical activity believed to be of benefit to the cardiovascular system.

Increased emphasis regarding the importance of establishing regular physical activity as a normal part of life in childhood and adolescence, and on developing interests in activities which can be carried into adulthood, are likely to be important influences on maintenance of appropriate body weight in adult life (see also page 137).

Genetic predisposition

It seems that it may be possible to predict adult obesity in young children if something is known about their family history. Studies of twins support a genetic predisposition to obesity. In other words, the pattern of distribution of fat and degree of obesity can be inherited. In a study of 40 000 subjects in the USA (Garn and Clark, 1976), the children of two lean partners were the thinnest and those of two obese parents were the fattest. However, the study was unable to exclude environmental influences.

The Danish Adoption Study has provided stronger evidence of a genetic component to obesity (Stunkard et al., 1986). There was a close relationship between the relative weight classification of the biological mother and her child but not between the mother who adopts and the adopted child. Studies among Pima Indians have also displayed familial aggregation of low levels of resting metabolic rate associated with an increased tendency to put on weight (Ravussin et al., 1988).

A large part of the familial tendency to obesity relates to energy intake, although differences in metabolic rate may also be a factor. The extent to which genetic or environmental factors are involved remains to be clarified, though the current view is that overeating is the major factor.

Yo-yo dieting and 'weight cycling'

There are those who can successfully lose weight but who cannot, or find it difficult to, maintain this weight loss. Such people may experience large swings in their weight over time, known as 'weight cycling', a phenomenon associated with yo-yo dieting. Weight regain after many weeks and months of struggling to slim can be very distressing and damaging to the self-esteem of patients, and weight cycling is suggested to be associated with an increased lack of control over food intake (the ability to sense hunger and satiety is disrupted). The rapid weight gain is often due to a return to previous and inappropriate eating habits, suggesting that more attention should be paid to supporting patients during the maintenance phase of weight management as well as during actual weight loss. The macronutrient composition of weight maintenance diets may be of particular importance (see page 137). Long-term follow-up and support may best be provided by groups (either slimming groups linked to the surgery or appropriate commercial ones).

Smoking and weight management

As a generalization, smokers have lower body weight than non-smokers and weight gain after giving up smoking is common. Those giving up smoking tend to snack more but there is also evidence of a decrease in resting metabolic rate, as well as an absence of the short-term thermogenic effects of smoking (Dallosso and James, 1984). Clients may give this as a reason for continuing to smoke. However, analysis of mortality data indicates that risks associated with smoking far outweigh those associated with a 10–15 kg rise in body weight (Royal College of Physicians, 1983).

Importance of physical activity

The contribution of physical activity and exercise to weight loss is frequently dismissed because of the enormous amount of energy that would need to be expended to counter the intake of energy from a meal or snack coupled with the stimulatory effect of mild exercise on appetite. However, this overlooks other ways in which exercise might affect total energy balance, such as via increased heat production and temporarily elevated metabolic rate, as well as its value in creating a feeling of well-being.

Garrow (1988) suggests that for those with only a few pounds to lose, probably the best method to effect weight loss (or weight maintenance) is an increase in physical activity. This alone can often be sufficient, in that it does not require a concomitant reduction in energy intake. The proviso to this is that there is no increase in energy intake in response to increased appetite associated with the higher activity level.

Since energy intake is not reduced, there is a greater chance that needs for essential nutrients will be met. Unbalanced slimming diets can readily provide inadequate levels of individual vitamins and minerals.

Who should be targeted for treatment?

A two-pronged approach to tackling weight

management will also of necessity involve treating established obesity. It is essential, however, that attempts to treat obesity are not half-hearted (Garrow, 1994), as without full commitment the chance of achieving worthwhile weight loss will be poor and the danger of further damaging the patient's self-esteem could be considerable, as will be the likelihood of inducing phenomena associated with weight cycling (see above). Indeed, Wooley and Garner (1994) suggest that, owing to poor success in treating obesity in the past, ineffective treatment for weight loss should be stopped. Instead, ways of reducing the medical and psychological costs of obesity by modifying risk factors for chronic disease should be considered, as well as helping patients to eat healthily, to exercise appropriately, to deal with the stigma associated with obesity and improve self-esteem, and to refrain from binge eating; however, trying to treat obesity itself should be abandoned.

Treatment goals might be: to stabilize eating patterns (and improve control of food intake), to improve dietary quality, to increase physical activity levels, to improve acceptance of body shape, and to aid management of stress.

Again action should be targeted, for example by directing attention to:

- **those who actually want to lose weight.** Potentially this could be a very large group and so the most effective approach is likely to be suitably structured slimming groups. There will always be a number of patients who fail to progress well with a group approach and who will need to be referred to specialist centres or clinics (see below).

- **children (over age 7 years) and adolescents** (see page 138).

- **those with medical problems known to be exacerbated by obesity** (for example diabetes, coronary heart disease, hypertension, osteoarthritis and a variety of disabilities).

- **women, between pregnancies, who have remained overweight after they have had their baby.** They are at risk of progressing to being obese and their child might also be at risk of becoming overweight through environmental influences in the home (see below).

Some have suggested that people with a high waist to hip ratio should be preferentially targeted for treatment (Ashwell, 1992). If a man has a waist to hip ratio above 1.00 or a woman has a value above 0.80, it is likely that there is a significantly higher risk of conditions such as heart disease and diabetes (see page 136).

Babies born to overweight or obese parents

There is an increased chance of a baby becoming overweight if it is born into a family with a tendency to obesity. It may therefore be worthwhile providing such parents with advice and support on weaning and feeding their child (and themselves), to help modify the environmental influences on energy intake to which the child will inevitably be subject. It is important that such advice is focused on the family rather than on the new baby or young child. In addition, if the mother put on excessive weight during the pregnancy, the advice could focus on reducing her body weight, once lactation is over.

Groups who should not be targeted

Some groups of obese people should **not** be targeted for advice on weight loss. These include: those who do not wish to lose weight (success is unlikely if the patient is not motivated), and pregnant and breast-feeding women.

The management of obesity in pregnant women has always been a controversial area. Whilst some obstetricians firmly believe that every effort should be made to prevent unnecessary weight gain in pregnancy, others believe that it is best not to impose restrictions. For further information on energy requirements and weight gain during pregnancy, see Chapter 1.

In addition, thought needs to be given to the advisability of treating obese elderly people who are otherwise healthy. Some would argue that they are best advised not to slim.

Opportunities and strategies for action

Some patients may voluntarily seek advice on diet and weight loss. In providing advice, various approaches can be taken by the practice team. The most appropriate strategy will vary from one patient to another, and a mixture of the following approaches are likely to be needed within the practice:

- one-to-one counselling, involving a dietitian or other appropriately trained professional

- surgery-based, clinic-based, or community-based slimming group

- referral to an appropriately structured, 'commercially' run slimming group, for example Weight Watchers

- referral to a leisure centre for a prescribed physical activity programme, although the benefits of this approach need to be evaluated (Iliffe et al., 1994).

In addition, patients can routinely be offered advice geared to preventing those who are already overweight progressing to obesity. For example, those patients (particularly young adults) encountered with a body mass index of, say, 28–30 could routinely be offered advice on weight management (diet, eating patterns and physical activity). In some cases, existing psychiatric problems need to be addressed before there is any real likelihood of sustainable weight loss being achieved, for example among persistent binge eaters. People with these problems need special psychiatric counselling to try and bring their eating habits back to normal and to improve their self-esteem. It may be more appropriate to move such people away from 'slimming' towards normal 'healthy eating'.

Dietary advice

A dietary regimen for weight reduction should:

- provide less energy than that required to maintain the body weight of the patient

- be nutritionally adequate

- be acceptable to the patient or, at least, tolerable.

Despite the complex aetiology of obesity and the proliferation of 'miracle cures', the concept of energy balance and maintenance of body weight can be refined to a simple equation. If energy intake exceeds energy expenditure, then the excess will accumulate as adipose tissue. To be successful, treatment for overweight and obesity must achieve a temporary negative energy balance so that fat stores can be burned to meet energy demands. This means that treatment must influence either the input of energy (diet), the output (exercise), or both. The suitability of different types of treatment for different levels of obesity are discussed in detail by Garrow (1988).

A major aim of treatment is to reduce body fat rather than lean tissue. Garrow suggests that if weight loss exceeds 1 kg/week, this could be at the expense of lean tissue. Loss of lean tissue has implications for metabolic rate because the level at which resting metabolic rate is set is determined by the quantity of lean tissue present. A fall in resting metabolic rate means that dietary energy requirements also fall and it becomes more difficult to sustain weight loss or to maintain weight at the desired level.

The recommended type of slimming diet is based on foods rich in essential nutrients but low in calories, chosen from the four main food groups — fruit and vegetables; bread, cereals and potatoes; milk and milk products; and lean meat and alternatives (see Appendix 1 and Part 1, page 31). Traditionally, the overall aim is to reduce energy intake to 1000–1500 kcal and to increase levels of physical activity. Increasingly these days, dietitians are experimenting with a more flexible approach in which energy reductions are often smaller, for example to 1500–2000 kcal, but in which compliance and subsequent sustained weight loss is often considerably improved (Frost et al., 1991).

Slimming aids can have a part to play in getting started, but in the long term it is important that appropriate eating habits are learned and this is best achieved by eating everyday foods.

Control of food intake

There are many physiological mechanisms which are believed to contribute to control of food intake in man. These are thought to be co-ordinated in part by the gastro-intestinal neuro-hormonal system and the hypo-thalamus.

There is some evidence to suggest that a brain neurotransmitter, serotonin (5-hydroxytryptamine) may have a key role in regulating both total food intake and the selection of carbohydrate-rich or protein-rich meals when there is a choice available. Altered 5-hydroxytryptamine levels may help explain pronounced craving and bingeing of carbohydrate-rich foods.

Although such behaviour may cause obesity in susceptible individuals, the main body of research does not support the existence of marked differences in eating behaviour between people who are overweight and those of normal weight.

Very low calorie diets

Very low calorie diets (VLCD) typically supply 600 kcal/day and are used for a period of days or weeks. Conventional eating is replaced by some kind of formula diet. Most recommend total meal replacement to start with, followed by partial substitution of meals later on. Very low calorie diets are designed to produce rapid weight loss.

In 1987, a working group of COMA, the government's Committee on Medical Aspects of Food Policy, reported on very low calorie diets following concern expressed on the basis of efficacy, safety and sales methods (DHSS, 1987). They advised that such diets should not be the preferred choice as a means of losing weight in obese people. In particular it was emphasized that they were not suitable for use by people with a relatively small amount of weight to lose. They also emphasized that very low calorie diets:

- are unsuitable for use by people who have: heart disease, kidney disease, hypertension, cancer and diabetes treated with insulin or sulphonylurea drugs; if this form of treatment is considered for people with these diseases, medical supervision under hospital conditions would be necessary

- are unsuitable for use by people who have porphyria and gout

- should be used under strict medical supervision with people who have: depression of more than a minor degree, schizophrenia, severe behaviour disorders, lithium therapy

- should never be used by women who are pregnant or breastfeeding, infants, children and adolescents or elderly people.

Very low calorie diets perhaps have a role in the severely obese or in those who have repeatedly failed to lose weight by conventional means, but they should never be used casually nor for longer than three to four weeks when they are the sole source of nutrition.

Tips on weight loss

The following are useful tips to give those trying to lose weight:

- Aim for a weight loss of 0.5–1.0 kg/week; this rate of loss is more likely to be permanent than faster rates.

- Good weight loss should be achieved on 1000 kcal/day (women) and 1200 kcal/day (men). Even a reduction to 1500 kcal/day will achieve gradual weight loss in most people, and is more likely to help compliance.

- Warn patients that weight loss may be rapid to begin with, but that this rate will probably tail off. This initial rapid weight loss is due to the loss of some glycogen and associated water, as well as adipose tissue. The rate of weight loss may slow down after this time when only adipose tissue is being lost. Acknowledgement of the change in the speed of weight loss may help prevent despondency and non-compliance.

- Set realistic goals, with a series of small targets which are attainable in the short term.

- Record weight once a week.

- Encouraging the patient to complete a food diary on a regular basis may increase awareness of what is being eaten.

- Allow treats — the opportunity to eat a favourite food once in a while can make all the difference to compliance.

- Although slimming aids can sometimes help, in general it is preferable if the daily slimming regimen comprises a wide variety of ordinary foods rich in essential nutrients, selected from each of the four main food groups (see Appendix 1).

- Build patients' confidence and help them to accept their own body image.

- Group support can be very effective.

- Many dieters reach a plateau and may have to reduce their energy intake further, sometimes temporarily, to continue weight loss.

- A complementary physical activity programme, tailored to the individual, is important. Not only does it expend some energy and improve well-being, it can also help tone the muscles as weight is being lost.

- With a reduction in energy intake, constipation can be a problem. Ensure that fibre and fluid intakes are adequate.

- Changes in energy intake, desire for food and specific cravings are known to occur at various stages of the menstrual cycle. This should be taken into account and discussed when planning a weight reduction programme. Fluid retention can also be a specific problem for some women.

- In some people, psychological factors make a considerable contribution to obesity. It can help to try to establish the patients' thoughts on why they are overweight.

- Give advice on maintaining new body weight once the desired weight loss has been achieved. Although strict restrictions on food intake may be lifted, if previous eating habits are adopted the person will probably regain the lost weight. A permanent change in food intake is usually necessary to maintain the lower weight.

- A good relationship between the dietitian/ doctor and the patient is paramount to successful weight loss and maintenance of the new body weight. Every attempt should be made to try to build up the self-esteem of patients who have not lost weight on follow-up and to attempt to establish the reasons for failure to do so.

Failure to lose weight

Many patients who are first referred for weight loss have inappropriate ideas about the foods that they should be eating to achieve weight loss. A diet of 1000 kcal is generally very restrictive compared to their usual intake. However, with good advice and patient motivation (see above), weight loss can be achieved.

There are also some patients who are well informed about what they should be eating and insist that they are sticking to the diet but do not lose weight. If the prognosis without weight loss is serious, further investigation is necessary. To establish whether the regimen is being adhered to, Garrow (1992) suggests that each day for 3–4 weeks the diet should consist solely of 2 pints of whole cows' milk (or the energy equivalent in semi-skimmed milk) and an unlimited intake of water [together with a multi-vitamin supplement with iron]. This regimen provides approximately 800 kcal. If weight loss is not achieved, referral to a specialist centre should be considered.

Management of underweight

Whilst considerable attention is paid to helping those who are overweight to slim, the plight of those who want to put on weight goes relatively unnoticed. Whilst advice can be given on maintaining weight, attempts to achieve weight gain by food supplements are often unsuccessful.

People who want to put on weight are best advised to select foods rich in starchy carbohydrate (such as bread, pasta, potatoes, rice) and foods which are good sources of essential nutrients, such as milk, lean meat, fruit and vegetables. Since the nutritional balance of their diet remains important, they should consume only moderate amounts of foods rich in fat and sugar and low in essential nutrients. Snacks during the day, based on wholesome foods, can be helpful.

Eating disorders

Some people, particularly adolescents and young adults, who present with low body weights may be suffering from an eating disorder such as anorexia nervosa or bulimia nervosa. For a review of these eating disorders, see Part 3, Eating Disorders.

References

Armstrong N et al. (1990) Patterns of physical activity among 11 to 16-year-old British children. *British Medical Journal* **301**, 203–5.

Ashwell M (1992) Obesity in middle aged women. In *Nutrition, Social Status and Health*. Proceedings of a National Dairy Council Conference 1991. London, National Dairy Council.

Bennett N et al. (1995) *Health Survey for England 1993*. Office of Population Censuses and Surveys. London, HMSO.

Bolton-Smith C and Woodward M (1993) The prevalence of overweight and obesity in different fat and sugar consumption groups. (Abstract only.) *Proceedings of the Nutrition Society* **52**, 383A.

Braddon REM et al. (1986) Onset of obesity in a 36 year birth cohort study. *British Medical Journal* **293**, 259–303.

Dallosso HM and James WPT (1984) The role of smoking in the regulation of energy balance. *International Journal of Obesity* **8**, 365–75.

DeCastro JM and Orozco S (1991) Moderate alcohol intake and spontaneous eating patterns of humans: evidence of unregulated supplementations. *American Journal of Clinical Nutrition* **52**, 246–53.

Department of Health, Committee on Medical Aspects of Food Policy (1991) *Dietary Reference Values for Food Energy and Nutrients for the United Kingdom. Report on Health and Social Subjects 41*. London, HMSO.

Department of Health and Social Security, Committee on Medical Aspects of Food Policy (1987) *The Use of Very Low Calorie Diets in Obesity. Report on Health and Social Subjects 13*. London, HMSO.

Flatt JP et al. (1985) Effects of dietary fat on postprandial substrate oxidation and on carbohydrate and fat balances. *Journal of Clinical Investigation* **76**, 1019–24.

Flatt JP (1987) The difference in the storage capacities for carbohydrate and for fat, and its implications in the regulation of body weight. *Annals of the New York Academy of Sciences* **499**, 104–23.

Frost G et al. (1991) A new method of energy prescription to improve weight loss. *Journal of Human Nutrition and Dietetics* **4**, 369–73.

Garn SM and Clark DC (1976) Trends in fatness and the origins of obesity. *Pediatrics* **57**, 442–56.

Garrow JS (1988) *Obesity and Related Diseases*. London, Churchill Livingstone.

Garrow JS (1991) Importance of obesity. *British Medical Journal* **303**, 704–6.

Garrow JS (1992) Treatment of obesity. *Lancet* **340**, 409–13.

Garrow JS (1994) Should obesity be treated? *British Medical Journal* **309**, 654–6.

Gregory J et al. (1990) *The Dietary and Nutritional Survey of British Adults*. Office of Population Censuses and Surveys. London, HMSO.

Health Education Authority (1991) *Enjoy Healthy Eating*. London, HEA.

Hill JO and Prentice AM (1995) Sugar and body weight regulation. *American Journal of Clinical Nutrition* **62** (suppl), 264S–274S.

Iliffe S et al. (1994) Prescribing exercise in general practice; look before you leap. *British Medical Journal* **309**, 494–5.

Jéquier E (1994) Carbohydrates as a source of energy. *American Journal of Clinical Nutrition* **59** (suppl), 682S–5S.

Larsson B et al. (1992) Is abdominal body fat distribution a major explanation for the sex difference in the incidence of myocardial infarction? *American Journal of Epidemiology* **135**, 266–73.

Prewitt TE et al. (1991) Changes in body weight, body composition, and energy intake in women fed high- and low-fat diets. *American Journal of Clinical Nutrition* **54**, 304–10.

Ravussin E et al. (1988) Reduced rate of energy

expenditure as a risk factor for body weight gain. *New England Journal of Medicine* **318,** 467–72.

Royal College of Physicians (1983) *Obesity*. London, Royal College of Physicians.

Sheppard J et al. (1991) Weight loss in women participating in a randomised trial of low-fat diets. *American Journal of Clinical Nutrition* **54,** 821–8.

Stunkard AJ et al. (1986) An adoption study of human obesity. *New England Journal of Medicine* **314,** 193–8.

Suter PM et al. (1992) The effect of ethanol on fat storage in healthy subjects. *New England Journal of Medicine* **326,** 983–7.

Tremblay A et al. (1991) Nutritional determinants of the increase in energy intake associated with a high-fat diet. *American Journal of Clinical Nutrition* **53,** 1134–7.

Volschenk PA et al. (1993) Evidence that fat oxidation is modulated by fat intake in lean but not obese women (Abstract only.) *Proceedings of the Nutrition Society* **52,** 310A.

White A et al. (1993) *Health Survey for England 1991*. Office of Population Censuses and Surveys. London, HMSO.

Wing R (1992) Changes in waist-hip ratio with weight loss and its association with change in cardiovascular risk factors. *American Journal of Clinical Nutrition* **55,** 1086–92.

Wooley SC and Garner DM (1994) Dietary treatments for obesity are ineffective. *British Medical Journal* **308,** 655–6.

Further reading

Buttriss J and Gray J (1993) *Obesity and Weight Management. Fact File 4*. London, NDC.

13

Dental health

Key points

1. Although the prevalence of dental caries has declined, it still remains a preventable disease. A reduction in consumption of non-milk extrinsic sugars (primarily sucrose) has been recommended, to an average intake of 11% of food energy.

2. Fluoride in the water supply, in toothpaste or applied topically is seen as the most effective anti-caries agent.

3. Dental caries is particularly prevalent in children. Babies should not be given sweetened drinks or bottle feeds with added sugar, and dummies should not be dipped in sweet drinks. With babies over six months, the use of a cup or lidded beaker should be encouraged to help prevent damage to emerging teeth. A cup or lidded beaker should largely replace a bottle by a year. Bottles — regardless of the contents — should never be left propped in babies' mouths. Promotion of healthy eating via playgroups and schools is important for older children.

4. Sugary foods and drinks should be discouraged.

5. Regular tooth brushing is important for the prevention of periodontal disease.

Dental caries

Although there has been a marked decline in the prevalence of dental caries in the UK (Hargreaves et al., 1987; Rugg-Gunn et al., 1988), it still remains a major preventable disease. Its prevalence is generally lower in London and South East England than in other regions of the UK and is higher in children from social classes 4 and 5 than in those from social classes 1 and 2 (Todd and Dodd, 1985). In 1987/88 the cost of the general dental services within the UK was £934.6 million, the majority being incurred in treating caries (DH, 1989).

Dental caries is a disease in which there is a complex interaction between host factors (the susceptibility of the tooth), dental plaque, dietary components and time. The evidence relating particular foods or food constituents to caries comes from many types of investigation including human epidemiological and observational studies, human intervention studies, animal experiments, *in vivo* measurements of plaque acidity, *in vivo* enamel slab experiments, and *in vitro* incubation experiments. Many of these investigations have shown a significant association between the level of sugar consumption and the prevalence and severity of dental caries. Diets containing high levels of starch but low levels of sugars are associated with a low incidence of caries (Russell et al., 1960; Kleemole-Kuyale and Rasaner, 1979). The Vipeholm Study (Gustafsson et al., 1954) showed that eating sugary foods between meals was associated with a markedly higher risk of dental caries than when sugar consumption was restricted to mealtimes.

Evidence suggests that intrinsic sugars (those integrated into the cellular structure of food), as in fruit, and the sugars found naturally in milk — lactose and galactose — are negligible causes of dental caries and are substantially less cariogenic than other sugars (Koulourides et al., 1976; Imfeld, 1983). Although fresh fruit appears to be of low cariogenicity, natural syrups such as honey, maple syrup, and concentrated fruit juices are cariogenic.

There is some indication that a few foods — cheese, milk and peanuts — may not only have a low capacity for producing caries but may also help prevent caries developing (Rugg-Gunn et al., 1975; Silva de A et al., 1986; O'Brien and O'Connor, 1993; Rugg-Gunn, 1993). The mechanisms proposed to explain this effect include an ability of these foods to raise the pH in the immediate vicinity of the tooth surface — either directly or by stimulating flow of saliva, which helps wash away the acid resulting from fermentation of sugars by plaque bacteria.

The COMA Report (DH, 1989) recommends that a reduction in the amount and frequency of consumption of non-milk extrinsic sugars (fruit juice, honey and 'added sugars'), principally sucrose, which in 1987 provided 14% of the average daily food energy supply in the UK, would be expected to reduce the prevalence of caries. Sucrose-rich foods should be replaced by fresh fruit, vegetables and starchy foods, such as rice, potatoes and bread. In support of this, the later COMA report on dietary reference values (DH, 1991) includes the advice that the average intake of non-milk extrinsic sugars should be reduced to 11% of food energy (see Part 1, page 7).

Fluoride

Fluoride has been shown to be the most effective agent for the prevention of caries and is at its most efficient when incorporated in water supplies and toothpaste (DH, 1989).

It is the topical action of fluoride on enamel and plaque which is now regarded as important. Topical fluoride or fissure sealants are recommended for physically handicapped children who find it difficult to brush their teeth. Children on special diets with an obligatory high sugar intake will also benefit from fissure sealants.

In the absence of water fluoridation, fluoride supplements in the form of drops or tablets taken on a daily basis can reduce caries levels in preschool children. Such supplements should not be started until six months of age and the dosage will depend on the concentration of fluoride in the drinking water

Table 13.1 *Supplemental fluoride dosage schedule (mg fluoride/day)*

Age of child	Concentration of fluoride in drinking water (ppm*)		
	<0.3	0.3–0.7	>0.7
6 months–2 years	0.25	0	0
2 years–4 years	0.50	0.25	0
Over 4 years	1.00	0.50	0

*ppm = parts per million.
Adapted from British Medical Association/Royal Pharmaceutical Society of Great Britain (1995).

(Table 13.1). It is important to inform parents about the level of local water fluoridation because the use of supplements should be discouraged if the drinking water is already fluoridated. The local water company or district dental officer should be able to provide information on the amount of fluoride that has been added to the drinking water.

At present there is no evidence that fluoridation of water at one part per million has had any negative long-term effects. There is no link between the addition of fluoride to water supplies and the incidence of, or mortality from, cancer (Knox, 1985).

At-risk groups

Dental caries can occur at any age but it is especially prevalent in preschool children (Table 13.2).

Alternatives to sugary foods and drinks

Suitable alternatives to sugary foods and drinks include:

- fresh fruit
- raw vegetables
- wholemeal bread sandwiches
- unsweetened yogurt or fromage frais
- wholegrain, low sugar breakfast cereal with milk

- unsalted nuts (these should not be given to children under five years of age because of the danger of choking)
- glass of milk
- cheese or cheese spread and crackers.

For healthy alternatives to sugary foods and drinks, and lunch box ideas, see Chapters 3 and 4.

Sweeteners

Non-sugar bulk sweeteners (sorbitol, isomalt, mannitol, xylitol and hydrogenated glucose syrup) and intense sweeteners (saccharin, aspartame, acesulfamine K and thaumatin) are virtually non-cariogenic. The Department of Health (1989) recommends that the greatest gain would be expected to occur if such sweeteners were used to replace sugars in foods ingested frequently, such as sweet snacks, drinks and liquid medicines.

Smoking and alcohol

Discussing dental health provides an opportunity to discourage smoking and heavy alcohol consumption. The nicotine from tobacco can cause staining of teeth, which can only be removed effectively by the dentist or hygienist (HEA, 1990a).

Table 13.2 *Guidelines for at-risk groups*

Infants and young children

- Sugars* should not be added to bottle feeds.

- Drinks should **never** be in contact with developing teeth for long periods. This relates to all drinks including herb teas and those containing natural fruit juices, hydrolysed corn starch and sugars.*

- Dummies or comforters should not be dipped in sugary* drinks.

- Bottles of milk, including breast milk, should not be left in a baby's mouth for long periods of time. In particular, they should not be left propped in a baby's mouth. Apart from damaging teeth, they can cause choking.

- To prevent damage to emerging teeth caused by sugars, the use of lidded beakers and plastic cups should be encouraged. These can be introduced at six months, and by one year of age they should have largely replaced the use of feeding bottles. The main reason for this recommendation is that it encourages children to take their drinks all in one go, rather than 'little and often'. This reduced frequency, particularly where sweetened drinks are concerned, helps to protect teeth.

- Parents sometimes give table sugar to babies to prevent or treat constipation. This is not a recommended practice.

Older children

- Promotion of healthy eating should occur in playgroups and schools both via nutrition education and by providing and encouraging sound food choices. (See page 147 for healthy alternatives to sugary foods and drinks.)

- Use of sugared* medicine should be restricted.

Elderly people

- Amount and frequency of non-milk extrinsic sugars should be reduced because teeth are more likely to decay owing to exposure of teeth roots and declining salivary flow.

---

*Sugars are soluble carbohydrates and are classified according to the number of saccharide units in their structure. Sucrose, which is a combination of the monosaccharides glucose and fructose, is the most widely used as a food. Other sugars commonly found in food and drinks, either naturally or added during manufacture, include glucose, fructose, lactose and maltose.

Smokers have more severe gum disease than non-smokers, and smoking is associated with oral cancer. Heavy alcohol consumption, particularly of spirits, has also been linked to oral cancer. When heavy drinking is combined with smoking there is a multiplicative effect (HEA, 1990b).

Periodontal disease

Periodontal disease, or peridontitis, leads to the loss of teeth in a large proportion of the adult population. It is due to the effect of dental plaque (a film of sugar, bacteria, and other mouth debris) on the gums which, if allowed to accumulate, becomes calcified and eventually forms deposits called calculus or tartar. When this occurs between the gum (gingiva) and the tooth, the gum can become infected. In the early stages of infection, the gums become inflamed (gingivitis) and may bleed. Gingivitis is reversible if the calculus is removed either by tooth brushing or clinical treatment. However, if it is neglected, the bacteria eventually invade the bone supporting the tooth resulting in loosening and finally loss of the tooth. Periodontal disease can develop slowly over a number of years, often without symptoms.

The amount of plaque and age of the person are by far the most important factors in the development of periodontal disease. In addition, other diseases, drugs and hormones can affect the periodontal tissue (Seymour and Heasman, 1992). There are few data available to draw any conclusions on the effects of most nutrients on periodontal disease (for review see Rugg-Gunn, 1993). Although there is strong evidence from animal studies that nutritional deficiencies have an adverse effect on periodontal tissues, this evidence is not yet substantiated in humans. Overall, periodontal tissues will benefit throughout life if good dietary practices are maintained. However, dietary supplementation of nutrients above levels accepted as adequate (see Part 1, Appendix 2), including supplementation with vitamin C, does not seem to improve periodontal health further.

The best way of maintaining periodontal health is regular and meticulous physical removal of plaque with an adequate toothbrush. Children should be taught from an early age to clean their teeth properly. A soft/medium textured multi-tufted nylon toothbrush is the most suitable type of brush to use, and brushing should take about 3 minutes. As long as all the surfaces of all the teeth are well cleaned, the exact method of brushing is not considered to be important.

References

British Medical Association/Royal Pharmaceutical Society of Great Britain (1995) *British National Formulary*. London, BMA/Pharmaceutical Press.

Department of Health, Committee on Medical Aspects of Food Policy (1989) *Dietary Sugars and Human Disease. Report on Health and Social Subjects 37*. London, HMSO.

Department of Health, Committee on Medical Aspects of Food Policy (1991) *Dietary Reference Values for Food Energy and Nutrients for the United Kingdom. Report on Health and Social Subjects 41*. London, HMSO.

Health Education Authority (1990a) *Give Your Mouth A Break*. London, HEA.

Health Education Authority (1990b) *Diet and Cancer: Briefing Paper*. London, HEA.

Gustafsson BE et al. (1954) The Vipeholm dental caries study: effect of different levels of carbohydrate intake on caries activity in 436 individuals observed for 5 years. *Acta Odontologica Scandinavica* **11**, 232–364.

Hargreaves JA et al. (1987) Changes in caries prevalence of Isle of Lewis children, a historical comparison from 1937 to 1984. *Caries Research* **21**, 277–84.

Imfeld TN (1983) *Identification of Low Caries Risk Dietary Components*. Basel, Karger.

Kleemole-Kuyale E and Rasaner L (1979) Dietary pattern of Finnish children with low and high caries experience. *Community Epidemical* **7**, 199–205.

Knox EG (1985) *Fluoridation of Water and Cancer: A Review of the Epidemiological Evidence. Report of the DHSS Working Party*. London, HMSO.

Koulourides T et al. (1976) Cariogenicity of nine sugars tested with an intra-oral device *in vivo*. *Caries Research* **10**, 427–41.

O'Brien NM and O'Connor TP (1993) Milk, cheese and dental caries. *Journal of the Society of Dairy Technology* **46**, 46–49.

Rugg-Gunn AJ et al. (1975) The effect of different meal patterns upon plaque pH in human subjects. *British Dental Journal* **139**, 351.

Rugg-Gunn AJ et al. (1988) Effect of fluoridation and secular trend in caries of 5 year old children living in Newcastle and Northumberland. *British Dental Journal* **165,** 359–64.

Rugg-Gunn AJ (1993) Dental caries — milk, cheese and other protective factors. In Rugg-Gunn AJ (Ed.) *Nutrition and Dental Health.* Oxford, OUP.

Russell AL et al. (1960) Dental surveys in relation to nutrition. *Public Health Report* **75,** 717–23.

Seymour RA and Heasman PA (1992) *Drug Diseases and the Peridontium.* Oxford, Oxford Medical Publications.

Silva MF de A et al. (1986) Effects of cheese on experimental caries in human subjects. *Caries Research* **20,** 263–9.

Todd JE and Dodd T (1985) Children's Dental Health in the United Kingdom 1983: a Survey carried out by the Social Survey Divisions of OPCS, on behalf of the United Kingdom Health Departments in collaboration with the Dental Schools in the Universities of Birmingham and Newcastle. London, HMSO.

Further reading

British Nutrition Foundation (1988) *The Role of Diet in Dental Health. Briefing Paper No 16.* London, BNF.

Buttriss J (1995) *Diet and Dental Health. Topical Update 5.* London, National Dairy Council.

Health Education Authority (1992) *A Handbook of Dental Health for Health Visitors.* London, HEA.

14

Food hygiene

Key points

1. The incidence of food poisoning has risen rapidly over the last decade; most cases are attributable to *Salmonella* species, *Listeria monocytogenes* and *Campylobacter jejuni*.

2. There are two main categories of food poisoning: (a) foodborne intoxication which usually results from the ingestion of toxins produced by bacteria in food is typically of rapid onset and short duration; (b) foodborne infection which is the result of ingestion of a food harbouring large numbers of bacteria is typically of later onset and longer duration.

3. Stricter attention to food hygiene is particularly important for vulnerable groups such as the ill and immuno-suppressed, the elderly, the very young and pregnant women, all of whom are at greatest risk of food poisoning.

4. Some foods carry a greater risk of bacterial contamination than others, for example short shelf-life foods which normally require chilled storage and are eaten cold or 'warmed up', poorly stored food which is reheated.

5. Particular guidance has been issued by the Department of Health with regard to listeriosis (pâté, mould-ripened soft cheese, cook-chill meals and ready-to-eat poultry) and salmonellosis (raw or partially cooked eggs, poultry and raw meat).

6. There is legislation covering food premises, retailers, and the food and catering industry to help prevent food poisoning and ensure a safer food supply for the consumer.

7. As a matter of routine, advice on basic food hygiene should be considered for families presenting regularly with diarrhoea suspected of being linked with food handling in the home (Appendix 2).

The number of food poisoning cases is increasing almost every year. Data provided by the Office of Population Censuses and Surveys (OPCS, personal communication) indicate that formal notifications have increased by more than 300% since 1980, and in 1989, a total of 38 086 cases were reported in England and Wales. Many experts believe that these figures represent just the tip of the iceberg and estimate that only 1 in 10 cases are ever reported.

Most of these increases are attributed to *Salmonella* species, in particular *S. enteriditis*, which now accounts for nearly half of all formal notifications, but sharp rises have also been seen in cases of listeriosis and campylobacter.

Food poisoning is the general term used to describe an acute disturbance of the gastro-intestinal tract that causes pain, diarrhoea, nausea and vomiting. Symptoms are often of relatively short duration. There are broadly two types of food poisoning: foodborne intoxication and foodborne infections.

Foodborne intoxications

Foodborne intoxications result from the ingestion of toxic substances, such as those produced by micro-organisms in foods, by naturally occurring toxins in foods or by chemical residues. The most common toxin-producing, food-poisoning bacteria are *Bacillus cereus*, *Staphylococcus aureus* and *Clostridium botulinum*. The incubation time for this type of food poisoning is usually relatively short, although *Clostridium botulinum* (the cause of botulism, which is extremely rare) can take up to 72 hours.

Bacillus cereus is capable of producing toxins in food which can cause vomiting or diarrhoea. They are not destroyed by reheating and are resistant even to laboratory autoclave temperatures. Spores may be found in cooked, reheated rice and other cereals and illness caused by these bacteria is often nicknamed the 'take-away syndrome', as they are common in refried rice (Table 14.1).

Staphylococcus aureus is another major cause of food poisoning. Symptoms include diarrhoea, nausea and vomiting and may last for 6–24 hours. The very young, elderly and ill are particularly vulnerable. These bacteria are present on the skin, in boils and the nose and throat of infected people and may be transferred to food during preparation by poor hygiene practices. They are destroyed by pasteurization and cooking but the spores are resistant up to 120°C. Cream cakes and cooked meats are high risk foods (Table 14.1).

Clostridium botulinum is fortunately a rare cause of poisoning but the disease can be fatal. All groups of people are vulnerable. It may be found in canned and bottled foods that have been inadequately sterilized or in damaged ('blown') cans. It can grow anaerobically, so the contents of cans are ideal breeding grounds. It requires very high temperatures, over 120°C, to be destroyed.

Foodborne infections

Foodborne infections, on the other hand, are of later onset and may take several days to resolve. They result from the ingestion of large numbers of bacteria in the food, such as *Salmonella* species, *Campylobacter jejuni*, *Escherichia coli*, *Listeria monocytogenes* or *Clostridium perfringens*. Once ingested, the bacteria establish themselves in the intestine and release their toxins. Normally the healthy body can cope with low level microbial con-

tamination and succumbs to their effects only when these micro-organisms obtain favourable growth conditions reaching very high numbers. However, susceptible groups such as the ill, the elderly and the very young are at risk at much lower levels of contamination.

Salmonella species may be found in uncooked poultry, meat and eggs. The government's Chief Medical Officer has advised the public to avoid raw eggs or uncooked foods made with them such as mayonnaise or mousse. The risk of harm to a healthy person is small, but vulnerable groups (elderly, ill, very young and pregnant women) are advised to consume eggs which have been cooked until both the white and yolk are solid. Symptoms of salmonellosis include stomach cramps, diarrhoea, nausea and vomiting and may last for up to a week. Salmonella is destroyed at about 70°C and the multiplication slowed below 5°C (Table 14.1).

Campylobacter jejuni is found in poultry and meat: undercooked chicken and inadequately barbecued meat present the greatest risks but heating to over 65°C kills the bacteria. The organism does not multiply in the food. Instead, it multiplies in the intestine after ingestion. Symptoms of campylobacter enteritis include diarrhoea and may last for 5–7 days or longer (Table 14.1).

Listeria monocytogenes can cause listeriosis. Symptoms range from fever and flu-like illness to meningitis and septicaemia and even death. It can cause miscarriage, stillbirth or severe illness in the newborn baby. Since February 1989 the government's Chief Medical Officer has advised pregnant women, young children, the elderly and those with suppressed immune systems to avoid eating certain mould-ripened soft cheeses (Camembert, Brie and blue vein varieties) and pâté. Other high risk foods include poultry, meat, raw (unpasteurized) milk, ready prepared salads and cook-chill foods. The bacteria can multiply slowly at refrigeration temperatures as low as 1°C and it is necessary, when cooking or re-heating foods, that the centre reaches at least 70°C (Table 14.1).

Table 14.1 *Common causes of food poisoning in Britain and related symptoms*

Contaminating micro-organisms	Causes	Symptoms
Salmonella species	Poor food hygiene practices — raw eggs, raw poultry, sausages and beef are improperly handled or inadequately cooked. Pet cat/dog or raw pet food can also be a source	Sudden and sometimes severe abdominal pain and diarrhoea lasting 1–3 days, often occurring within 16–48 hours of consuming the food. After an attack, the bacteria can continue to be excreted in faeces for up to six weeks
Campylobacter jejuni	Poultry and raw meat, unpasteurized milk and infected pets (about 50% of dogs and cats excrete the bacteria in their faeces, and their coats can become infected)	In young children, the bacteria may cause mild diarrhoea but in older children and adults, the symptoms are more protracted. Symptoms typically appear in 16–48 hours and may include fever, headache and backache, aching limbs, abdominal pains and nausea. This is followed by severe diarrhoea which may be bloodstained and can last up to two weeks
Staphylococcus aureus	These bacteria can multiply at room temperature in contaminated foods such as custards, cream, cakes and trifles, cooked meat and poultry dishes and seafood such as prawns. As the bacteria can be carried on human skin, personal hygiene when handling these foods is especially important	Symptoms are similar to salmonella poisoning (vomiting can be profuse) and usually occur within a few hours (1–6) of eating the food and may last for 6–24 hours
Bacillus cereus	Common food vehicles include cooked rice and pasta, cooked meat and poultry, meat products, soups, sauces and vegetables	Two types of response to contamination are found: nausea and vomiting 1–5 hours, usually after eating boiled or fried rice dishes; abdominal pain and diarrhoea 4–16 hours after eating a variety of other foods (usually subsides in 12–24 hours)
Clostridium perfringens	These bacteria grow very rapidly in warm foods, particularly cooked meat dishes. Contamination can be avoided by rapid cooling of cooked dishes which are to be stored, and thorough reheating	Symptoms are relatively mild — profuse diarrhoea and acute abdominal pain. Fever and nausea are relatively rare
Listeria monocytogenes	Most people exposed to this organism do not become ill. Those most at risk are pregnant women, new babies, elderly people and those with a suppressed immune system. Foods in which small numbers of bacteria have been found include pâté, raw chicken, cook-chill food, soft mould-ripened cheeses, and pre-packed salads. Unusually, the bacteria can grow at low temperatures	Symptoms of listeriosis include fever, septicaemia and meningitis and these can lead to spontaneous abortion

Hepatitis or inflammation of the liver can also result from poor food handling practices. Hepatitis A (infectious hepatitis) is transmitted via an anal–oral cycle, and is characterized by an incubation period of 15–50 days. It causes a debilitating, low mortality disease that sometimes includes jaundice. Shellfish are the most common cause, presumably because they grow in waters which are increasingly subject to human faecal pollution and are able to collect the virus from the water via their filter-feeding activities. However, many other foods subject to handling by an infected person can also serve as a vehicle.

Other types of food poisoning can be caused by moulds and viruses. Some moulds produce mycotoxins which can result in serious illness if a contaminated food is eaten. Viruses can be introduced into food through faecal contamination by food handlers or via contaminated water. Shellfish is the most common cause of viral infection.

High risk foods

Almost all categories of food are potential sources of bacteria and the risk of food poisoning is increased in those whose immune system is compromised. The foods carrying the greatest risk of contamination with bacteria and hence causing food poisoning are those which readily support the growth of harmful bacteria and are also likely to be eaten uncooked or with only minimal heat treatment. Therefore short shelf-life foods which normally require chilled storage and are eaten cold or only 'warmed up', carry the highest risk. Foods which have been re-contaminated and poorly stored after cooking also pose a health risk. These high risk foods include:

- meat, poultry, fish, shellfish and dishes containing them, especially if they are inadequately cooked or if they are cooked, stored and then inadequately reheated

- meat products including burgers, pâté, gravy and stock

- uncooked or lightly cooked eggs and products made from uncooked or lightly cooked eggs (e.g. mayonnaise)

- soft mould-ripened cheeses, unpasteurized milk and cream and dishes containing them, artificial cream

- cooked rice.

Preventing food poisoning

Food Safety Act 1990

The Food Safety Act 1990, which came into force on 1 January 1991, is designed to ensure a safer food supply for the public. It lays down strict hygiene legislation for food premises, food handlers and retailers, enforcement regulations and consumer protection. For example, it requires that all food handlers have appropriate food hygiene training. Under this Act it is an offence to sell or supply food which does not meet food safety requirements. It gives authority to enforcement officers (usually environmental health officers) to issue improvement notices where a food business does not meet the food hygiene requirements and allows them to close down any business which poses an imminent health risk.

Food Hygiene (Amendment) Regulations 1990

These regulations, which came into force in April 1991, introduced a system of temperature controls for certain foods throughout the food chain so as to contain the growth of harmful micro-organisms. They specify two temperature brackets for perishable foods. Ready meals and other prepared foods have to be kept at a temperature no higher than 8°C. Foods particularly at risk, including cut, mould-ripened soft cheeses, cooked meats, ready prepared salads and pâtés, have to be kept at or below 5°C.

Practical guidelines on food quality and safety, food control systems and operational factors that implement the legislation contained in the Food Safety Act 1990 are covered in *Guidelines to Good Catering*

Practice published by the Institute of Food Science and Technology (1992).

The Food Safety Directorate (Ministry of Agriculture, Fisheries and Food) as well as a number of food retailers have published guidelines on safe food handling for the public. These give practical advice on hygienic shopping, storage, food preparation and cooking.

The guidelines in Appendix 2 can be used when advising on food hygiene for those at particular risk of food poisoning, for example pregnant women, young children, the elderly and those with a compromised immune system due to illness.

Travellers' diarrhoea

A wide range of parasitic infestations can be contracted whilst travelling abroad, especially in underdeveloped countries. But people travelling from one country to another (even within Europe) often experience diarrhoea which is not caused by pathogenic organisms but is triggered by exposure to differences in the types and environmental concentrations of non-pathogenic micro-organisms or perhaps by differences in diet. Adaptation after a few days frequently occurs and personal hygiene or food-handling practices are often not at fault. However, if bouts of diarrhoea and sickness occur regularly within a family, poor hygiene may be a factor, particularly if the family has not recently travelled. It is important that genuine cases of food poisoning are notified; under-reporting is thought to be common currently.

Reference

Institute of Food Science and Technology (1992) *Guidelines to Good Catering Practice.* London, IFST.

Further reading

British Nutrition Foundation (1989) *How Safe is Our Food? BNF Nutrition Bulletin* **14**.

Donaldson RJ (1988) *Essential Food Hygiene.* London, Royal Society of Health.

Fox BA and Cameron AG (1989) *Food Science, Nutrition and Health.* 5th edn. Sevenoaks, Hodder & Stoughton.

Institution of Environmental Health Officers (1991) *The Food Hygiene Handbook.* 6th edn. South Yorkshire, Highfield Publications.

Kipps M (1991) Food poisoning. *Nutrition and Food Science*, May/June, pp 19–21.

Useful leaflets

Domestos Advisory Service. *Wise up to Food Hygiene.* Domestos Advisory Service, 114 Cromwell Road, London SW7 4ES.

Ministry of Agriculture, Fisheries and Food (1991) *Food Safety.* Ref: PB0551. Foodsense, London SE99 7TT (Tel: 01645 556 000).

Ministry of Agriculture, Fisheries and Food (1994) *Keeping Food Cool and Safe.* Ref: PB1649. Foodsense, London SE99 7TT (Tel: 01645 556 000).

St Ivel (1994) *Enjoying Food at its Best* (FS/05/94) Nutrition and Consumer Services, St Ivel House, Interface Business Park, Wootton Bassett, Swindon, Wiltshire SN4 8QE (Tel: 01793 848 444).

Appendices

APPENDIX 1

The Balance of Good Health

The new National Food Guide, *The Balance of Good Health*, has been developed to help health professionals provide people with a consistent and practical message about healthy eating. An aim of the Guide is to help reduce the confusion about what healthy eating really means. It demonstrates that people do not have to give up the foods they most like for the sake of their health. Variety within the diet is of particular importance and snacks as well as meals count towards the healthy balance.

The size of the divisions within the 'plate' shows the balance of foods which should be consumed to achieve a good healthy diet, with more emphasis being given to the Bread, other cereals and potatoes group and to the Fruit and vegetables group (Figure A1). In contrast to the four largest groups, foods in the fifth group — Fatty and sugary foods — are not essential to a healthy diet but add choice and palatability. It is not necessary to achieve this balance at every meal or even every day, but the balance should be achieved over the period of a week or so.

This new initiative has been developed under the auspices of the Health of the Nation initiative and is consistent with the information on selecting a healthy and balanced diet provided in detail in Part 1, on page 31.

The Balance of Good Health is based on the Government's Eight Guidelines for a Healthy Diet:

- Enjoy your food
- Eat a variety of different foods
- Eat the right amount to be a healthy weight
- Eat plenty of foods rich in starch and fibre
- Don't eat too much fat
- Don't eat sugary foods too often
- Look after the vitamins and minerals in your food
- If you drink alcohol, keep within sensible limits.

The Balance of Good Health applies to most people, including vegetarians, people who need to lose weight and people of all ethnic origins. It does not apply to children under the age of two who need whole milk and full fat dairy products (see Chapters 2 and 3).

Copies of a leaflet for health professionals to support *The Balance of Good Health* can be obtained from local health promotion units and departments.

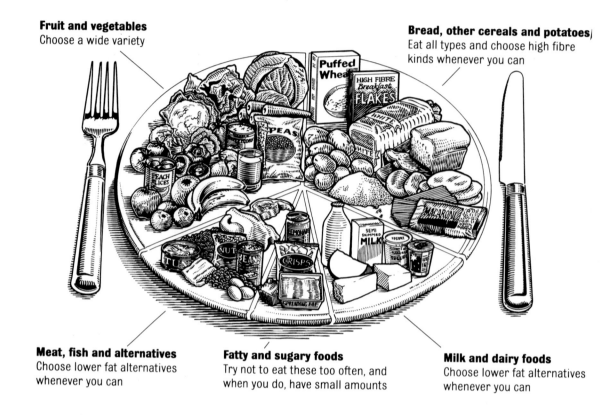

Fruit and vegetables
Choose a wide variety

Bread, other cereals and potatoes
Eat all types and choose high fibre
kinds whenever you can

Meat, fish and alternatives
Choose lower fat alternatives
whenever you can

Fatty and sugary foods
Try not to eat these too often, and
when you do, have small amounts

Milk and dairy foods
Choose lower fat alternatives
whenever you can

Figure A1 *The Balance of Good Health.*

Source: Health Education Authority (1994) *The Balance of Good Health. National Food Guide.* London, HEA.
Reproduced with permission.

Hygiene rules for the kitchen

The following advice should be considered for all families who present regularly with diarrhoea which is suspected to be related to food handling. It may be useful to photocopy these sections and use them as a hand-out for such patients.

Cleanliness in the kitchen

1. Keep all working surfaces scrupulously clean.

2. Wash all utensils and chopping boards after they have come into contact with raw meat, poultry or eggs, to prevent cross-contamination with foods that will not be cooked. Use separate, easily identified chopping boards for foods which are to be cooked, for example raw meat.

3. Keep kitchen cloths clean. It is often more hygienic to rinse crockery in hot water after washing up, and allow to dry, than to wipe it with a tea towel which is not absolutely clean. Use kitchen paper to mop up spills and to clean surfaces, rather than a dish cloth.

4. Keep waste bins covered and away from food. Clean them regularly with disinfectant.

5. Keep pets off work surfaces and away from food.

Hygienic food handling

1. Cook meat thoroughly to destroy bacteria. Do not eat under-cooked poultry or meat products.

2. Cool cooked foods as quickly as possible, if they are to be stored.

3. Always keep food covered and do not leave it standing around in the kitchen.

4. Store food in a cool place, preferably a refrigerator. (The coldest part of domestic refrigerators should operate at or below 5°C and be checked from time to time.) Keeping a fridge thermometer in the fridge is a good idea.

5. Store eggs in a refrigerator when possible.

6. Never overload the fridge as this can reduce circulation of cool air.

7. If storing raw and cooked foods together, keep the cooked above the raw so that blood or possibly contaminated fluids cannot drip onto cooked food and re-contaminate it.

8. Wash all food thoroughly (preferably under running water), especially salads, fruit and vegetables which will be eaten raw.

9. The colder chilled foods are kept between purchase and storage at home, the better. Make sure cooked-chilled meals are re-heated thoroughly and according to instructions.

10. When re-heating food, make sure it is heated until piping hot all the way through and do not reheat more than once.

11. When using a microwave to reheat food, observe the standing times recommended by the manufacturer to ensure the food attains an even temperature before it is eaten.

12. Keep foods (especially fresh meat and fish) for as short a time as possible, follow storage instructions and do not keep foods beyond their 'use by' or 'best before' dates.

Personal hygiene

1. Always wash hands before preparing food, after visiting the toilet, and after emptying the rubbish bin.

2. Never lick fingers or utensils and put them back into food.

3. Wash hands after blowing your nose while handling food.

4. Keep nails clean and hair out of food.

5. Do not handle the food you are preparing if you have a heavy cold, sickness or diarrhoea.

6. Wear a clean apron.

7. Cover all cuts, spots and pimples, particularly on the hands, with a waterproof dressing and replace it often.

Source: Buttriss J (Ed.) (1995) *Nutrition in General Practice*. Part 2: *Promoting Health and Preventing Disease*. London, Royal College of General Practitioners.

COLLEGE PUBLICATIONS

REPORTS FROM GENERAL PRACTICE	*Members*	*Non-Members*
18–21. Combined Reports on Prevention	£9.00	£9.90
22. Healthier Children—Thinking Prevention	£5.50	£6.05
23. What Sort of Doctor?	£5.00	£5.50
24. Alcohol—a Balanced View	£5.00	£5.50
25. The Front Line of the Health Service	£5.00	£5.50
26. The Development and Implementation of Clinical Guidelines ...	£10.00	£11.00

BOOKS AND BOOKLETS

The Future General Practitioner—Learning and Teaching	£9.50	£10.45
A History of the Royal College of General Practitioners	£10.00	£11.00
RCGP Members' Reference Book	£20.00	£20.00
Epidemiology in Country Practice	£15.00	£16.50
Will Pickles of Wensleydale	£10.50	£11.55
Handbook of Preventive Care for Preschool Children (2nd edn)	£5.00	£5.50
Trends in General Practice Computing	£12.50	£13.75
In Pursuit of Quality	£15.00	£16.50
Sir James Mackenzie MD	£12.50	£13.75
Prevention and the Primary Care Team	£3.00	£3.30
14 Prince's Gate. Home of the Royal College of General Practitioners	£8.50	£9.35
To Heal or to Harm. The Prevention of Somatic Fixation in General Practice	£12.50	£13.75
Doctors Talking to Patients	£10.50	£11.55
Family Medicine—The Medical Life History of Families	£15.00	£16.50
Milestones—The Diary of a Trainee GP	£9.95	£10.95
The Longest Art	£15.00	£16.50
The Writings of John Hunt	£55.00	£60.50
Balancing Dreams and Discipline—The Manager in Practice	£13.50	£14.85
Partnership with Patients	£6.00	£6.60
Forty Years On (The History of the College)	£18.00	£20.00
Counting on Quality	£13.50	£14.85
The MRCGP Examination	£15.00	£16.50
RCGP/CRMF GP Palliative Care Facilitator Project	£12.00	£13.20
Psychiatry in General Practice	£15.00★	£16.50★
Psychiatry and General Practice Today	£17.50★	£17.50★

★These two books can be bought together for £29.

These publications can be obtained from the Sales Office, Royal College of General Practitioners, 14 Princes Gate, Hyde Park, London SW7 1PU (Tel: 0171-823 9698). Prices include postage. Access and Visa are welcome (Tel: 0171-225 3048).

COLLEGE PUBLICATIONS

OCCASIONAL PAPERS

	Members	Non-Members
4. A System of Training for General Practice (2nd edn) … … … … …	£7.50	£8.25
25. Social Class and Health Status: Inequality or Difference … … … … …	£3.50	£3.85
27. Clinical Knowledge and Education for General Practice … … … … …	£3.50	£3.85
28. Undergraduate Medical Education in General Practice … … … … …	£3.50	£3.85
30. Priority Objectives for General Practice Vocational Training (2nd edn) …	£3.50	£3.85
31. Booking for Maternity Care: A Comparison of Two Systems … … …	£3.50	£3.85
32. An Atlas of Bedside Microscopy … … … … … … … … … …	£8.50	£9.35
33. Working Together—Learning Together … … … … … … … …	£3.00	£3.30
34. Course Organizers in General Practice … … … … … … … … …	£4.50	£4.95
35. Preventive Care of the Elderly: A Review of Current Developments … …	£5.00	£5.50
36. The Presentation of Depression: Current Approaches … … … … …	£7.50	£8.25
38. Continuing Education for General Practitioners … … … … … … …	£5.00	£5.50
39. Practice Assessment and Quality of Care … … … … … … … …	£7.50	£8.25
40. Rating Scales for Vocational Training in General Practice 1988 … … …	£5.00	£5.50
41. Practice Activity Analysis … … … … … … … … … … … …	£7.50	£8.25
42. The Contribution of Academic General Practice to Undergraduate Medical Education … … … … … … … … … …	£6.50	£7.15
43. Community Hospitals—Preparing for the Future … … … … …	£8.50	£9.35
44. Towards a Curriculum for General Practice Training … … … … …	£6.00	£6.60
45. Care of Old People: A Framework for Progress … … … … … …	£7.00	£7.70
46. Examination for Membership of the Royal College of General Practitioners	£6.50	£7.15
47. Primary Care for People with a Mental Handicap … … … … …	£7.50	£8.25
48. The Interface Study … … … … … … … … … … … … …	£7.50	£8.25
49. A College Plan—Priorities for the Future … … … … … … … …	£9.50	£10.45
50. Fellowship by Assessment (2nd edn) … … … … … … … … …	£15.00	£16.50
51. Higher Professional Education Courses in the United Kingdom … …	£6.50	£7.15
52. Interprofessional Collaboration in Primary Health Care Organizations …	£6.50	£7.15
53. Annual and Seasonal Variation in the Incidence of Common Diseases …	£6.50	£7.15
54. Prescribing in General Practice … … … … … … … … … … …	£7.50	£8.25
55. Guidelines for the Measurement of Hyperlipidaemia in General Practice	£6.00	£6.60
56. The European Study of Referrals from Primary to Secondary Care … …	£7.50	£8.25
57. Planning Primary Care … … … … … … … … … … … … …	£9.00	£9.90
58. Clinical Guidelines—Report of a Local Initiative … … … … …	£11.00	£12.10
59. Health Checks for People Aged 75 and Over … … … … … … …	£9.00	£9.90
60. Report of a Joint Working Group on Shared Care … … … … …	£6.00	£6.60
61. Stress Management in General Practice … … … … … … … … …	£9.00	£9.90
62. The Application of a General Practice Database to Pharmaco Epidemiology	£10.00	£11.00
63. Portfolio-based Learning in General Practice … … … … … … …	£9.00	£9.90
64. Community Participation in Primary Care … … … … … … … …	£9.00	£9.90
65. What is Good General Practice? … … … … … … … … … … …	£10.00	£11.00
66. Report of the Inner City Task Force of the Royal College of General Practitioners … … … … … … … … … … … … … …	£10.00	£11.00
67. Shared Care for Diabetes … … … … … … … … … … … …	£9.00	£9.90
68. Influences on Computer Use in General Practice … … … … … …	£15.00	£16.50
69. Drug Education in General Practice … … … … … … … … …	£12.00	£13.20
70. Significant Event Auditing … … … … … … … … … … … …	£15.00	£16.50
71. Rural General Practice in the United Kingdom … … … … … …	£10.00	£11.00

These publications can be obtained from the Sales Office, Royal College of General Practitioners, 14 Princes Gate, Hyde Park, London SW7 1PU (Tel: 0171-823 9698). Prices include postage. Access and Visa are welcome (Tel: 0171-225 3048).

COLLEGE PUBLICATIONS

CLINICAL SERIES

	Members	Non-Members
*Asthma in Practice	£12.50	£13.75
*Back Pain in General Practice	£9.00	£9.90
Coronary Heart Disease	£6.00	£6.60
*Cot Death	£6.00	£6.60
*Counselling in General Practice	£8.50	£9.35
*Depression	£8.50	£9.35
*Diabetes in General Practice	£12.50	£13.75
*Epilepsy	£7.50	£8.25
*Hormone Replacement Therapy	£12.00	£13.20
*Hypertension	£4.50	£4.95
*Incontinence	£14.00	£15.40
Minor Surgery in General Practice	£13.00	£14.30
*Motor Neurone Disease	£6.00	£6.60
Multiple Sclerosis	£14.00	£15.40
*Nutrition in General Practice		
1 Basic Principles of Nutrition	£8.50	£9.35
2 Promoting Health and Preventing Disease	£15.00	£16.50
Parkinson's Disease	£7.00	£7.70
Rheumatoid Arthritis	£14.00	£15.40
Schizophrenia	£12.00	£13.20
Terminal Care	£13.00	£14.30

PRACTICE ORGANIZATION SERIES

	Members	Non-Members
Age/Sex Registers	£3.00	£3.30
Appointment Systems	£5.00	£5.50
Entering General Practice	£6.00	£6.60
*Health and Safety at Work	£15.00	£16.50
Management Appreciation	£17.50	£19.25
Practice Information Booklets	£6.00	£6.60
Practice Profile	£13.50	£15.00

*Book format. The remaining titles are in folder format.

VIDEO PACKAGES

Management in Practice	£19.50
Additional course books	£4.50
Partnerships–Can We Talk?	£45.00
We Need a Practice Manager	£24.95
Additional course books	£6.50
Who Killed Susan Thompson?	£30.00
Additional course books	£5.00

These publications can be obtained from the Sales Office, Royal College of General Practitioners, 14 Princes Gate, Hyde Park, London SW7 1PU (Tel: 0171-823 9698). Prices include postage. Access and Visa are welcome (Tel: 0171-225 3048).